SUGAR FREE . . .

MICROWAVERY

SUGAR FREE . . .

MICROWAVERY

By Judith Soley Majors

Cover design and illustrations
by Charles B. Wells

BALLANTINE BOOKS • NEW YORK

To JACK and CARRIE
whose gentle and loving spirit lives in all my books
and will always be in my heart.

Library of Congress Catalog Card Number: 90-93517

ISBN: 0-345-36788-X

Cover design and illustrations by Charles B. Wells

Manufactured in the United States of America

First Ballantine Books Edition: May 1991

10 9 8 7 6 5 4 3 2 1

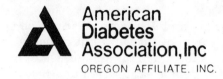

American
Diabetes
Association, Inc
OREGON AFFILIATE. INC.

3607 S.W. Corbett   Portland. Oregon 97201   (503) 228-0849

April 18, 1980

"Sugar Free....Microwavery"

With the blessing and the approval
of the
Dietetic Committee
American Diabetes Association, Inc.
Oregon Affiliate, Inc.

Rita Dewart

Rita Dewart
Executive Director

Moving Forward:

The microwave and diet were meant to be partners! The quickness and ease of preparation take much of the work out of being on a special diet and the microwave eliminates the need for much fat and grease in cooking thus cutting the calories considerably! Some people eat to live but I live to eat and have found diabetes does not rob me of one bit of pleasure and my microwave enhances many recipes. Armed with the exchange list and files of favorite recipes, many mine and many shared by friends, I set out to convert to microwave legal foods, in legal amounts, to be most appetizing, enjoyable, quick and economical.

Along the way there have been some failures (some so bad even Alice, the dog, declined to sample), many successes, a sampling of which are shared in this book. The dishes are for the whole family to enjoy, and are not diet-like and I am sure they will be enjoyed not only by persons on a special diet but by any individual who wants to eat well and stay healthy!

JUDY MAJORS

With much heartfelt thanks:
OREGON DIABETES ASSOCIATION, INC.
BARBARA VERHOFF BILLETTE, RD, professional guidance and friendship
VICKY HUTCHINSON, encouragement, recipe sharing and friendship
RITA DEWART, encouragement and invaluable support
MY FAMILY, sampling, patience, understanding and continual support
MY MOM AND DAD, manuscript preparation and sampling
MY FRIENDS, recipe sharing and testing

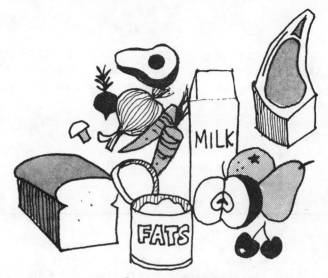

BASIC EXCHANGE LIST

EXCHANGE PROGRAM

The exchange program offers a variety of food to fit each individual likes and needs in specific amounts. By using the six exchange lists and foods in specified numbers and amounts to fit your diet, you can create a variety of taste sensations and almost forget you're on a diet!

The exchange program is simply a trade of one food for another in a specific food group for a food that is nearly equal in calories, carbohydrates, protein and fat. Also foods in each exchange group have similar mineral and vitamin content.

A well balanced diet consists of foods from each food group, as no single exchange group can supply all the nutrients our body requires for good health.

The energy value of food is expressed by the calorie count. The primary energy sources are fats, proteins and carbohydrates. Sugars and starches are the most common carbohydrates. The foods in the following exchange lists work together to provide the necessary nutrients that are essential to body function.

The real trick is to carefully measure the amounts of food used. All amounts are given in household measurement and are based on the ''new'' ADA exchange lists.

FREE EXCHANGES

These foods and seasonings contain negligible amounts of protein, fat or carbohydrate and may be used in unlimited amounts:

Diet type (calorie free) beverages
Coffee
Tea
Horseradish
Unsweetened pickles (try our prize
   winning dill pickles)
Raw lettuce
Unsweetened gelatin
Salt and pepper
Garlic
Celery salt
Radishes
Lemon juice
Lime juice

Paprika
Parsley
Mustard
Onion powder and salt
Vinegar
Cinnamon and Nutmeg
Fat free bouillon
Fat free consomme
Unsweetened cranberries
Mint
Herbs
Soy sauce
Non-calorie sweeteners

LIST 1: MILK EXCHANGES
Non-Fat, Low-Fat and Whole Milk

Each milk exchange contains 12 grams of carbohydrate, 8 grams of protein, a negligible amount of fat and 80 calories.

Non-Fat Fortified Milk
Skim or non-fat milk	1 cup
Powdered non-fat milk (dry)	1/3 cup
Canned evaporated skim milk	1/2 cup
Skim type buttermilk	1 cup
Unflavored yogurt (from skim milk)	1 cup

Low-Fat Fortified Milk
1% fat fortified milk (omit 1/2 fat exchange)	1 cup
2% fat fortified milk (omit 1 fat exchange)	1 cup
Unflavored yogurt from 2% fortified milk (omit 1 fat exchange)	1 cup

Whole Milk (omit 2 fat exchanges for each)
Whole milk	1 cup
Evaporated canned whole milk	1/2 cup
Buttermilk made from whole milk	1 cup
Unflavored yogurt (made from whole milk)	1 cup
Ice milk	1 cup

Milk is the leading source of calcium. It also contains protein, phosphorus, B-vitamins, magnesium and vitamins A and D. The milk exchange may be used to drink or included in recipes or added to cereal, coffee or other foods as desired. Remember to count the amount of milk added to other foods.

LIST 2: VEGETABLE EXCHANGES

Each vegetable exchange contains approximately 5 grams of carbohydrate, 2 grams of protein and 25 calories.
• One exchange equals $1/2$ cup unless noted.

Artichoke (1)	Chilies	Onions
Asparagus	Collards	Rhubarb
Bean Sprouts	Cucumber	Rutabagas
Beets	Dandelion	Sauerkraut
Broccoli	Eggplant	Spinach
Brussels Sprouts	Green Beans (String)	Squash (summer)
Cabbage	Green Pepper	Tomatoes
Carrots	Kale	Tomato Juice
Cauliflower	Mushrooms	Turnips
Celery	Mustard Greens	V-8 Juice
Chard	Okra	Zucchini

The following vegetables may be used raw as desired. Calories negligible.

Alfalfa Sprouts　　　　　　　　Lettuce
Chicory　　　　　　　　　　　　Onion Tops (green)
Chinese Cabbage　　　　　　　　Parsley
Chives　　　　　　　　　　　　Radishes
Endive　　　　　　　　　　　　Watercress
Escarole

• Check the bread exchange list for starchy vegetables.
Vegetables are rich sources of vitamins, and fiber is present in all vegetables.

LIST 3: FRUIT EXCHANGES

Each fruit exchange contains 10 grams of carbohydrate and 40 calories.
Fruits may be used fresh, dried, cooked, frozen, canned or raw as long as there are no sugars added.

Fruit	Amount	Fruit	Amount
Apple	1 small	Grape Juice	$1/4$ cup
Apple Juice	$1/3$ cup	Honeydew Melon	$1/8$ medium
Apple sauce (sugar free)	$1/2$ cup	Mango	$1/2$ small
Apricots (fresh or dried)	2 (4 halves)	Nectarine	1 small
Banana	$1/2$ small	Orange	1 small
Berries:		Orange Juice	$1/2$ cup
Blackberries	$1/2$ cup	Papaya	$3/4$ cup
Blueberries	$1/2$ cup	Peach	1 medium
Cranberries (sugar free)	Free exchange	Pear	1 small
Raspberries	$1/2$ cup	Pineapple	$1/2$ cup
Strawberries	$3/4$ cup	Pineapple Juice	$1/3$ cup
Cantaloupe	$1/4$ small	Plums	2 medium
Cherries	10 large	Pomegranate	1 small
Cider	$1/3$ cup	Prunes	2 medium
Dates	2	Prune Juice	$1/4$ cup
Figs	1	Raisins	2 tablespoons
Grapefruit	$1/2$	Tangelo	1 small
Grapefruit Juice	$1/2$ cup	Tangerine	1 medium
Grapes	12 large		

Fruits supply fiber, various amounts of vitamins A and C, folacin and potassium.

LIST 4: BREAD EXCHANGES
(Breads, cereals, crackers and starchy vegetables)

Each bread exchange contains 15 grams of carbohydrate, 2 grams of protein and 70 calories.

Breads	Amount	Crackers	Amount
Bagel	1/2 small	Arrow root	3
Pumpernickel	1 slice	Graham	2 2$^{1}/_{2}$″ square
Rye Bread	1 slice	Oyster	20
Raisin	1 slice	Pretzels	25 3$^{1}/_{2}$″ long
White (incl. French)	1 slice		× $^{1}/_{8}$″ dia.
Whole wheat	1 slice	Rye Krisp	3
Popover	1	Saltines	6
English Muffin	1/2 small	Soda Crackers	4
Plain roll (bread type)	1		
Hot dog bun	1/2		
Hamburger bun	1/2		
Croutons	1/2 cup plain		
Dried bread crumbs	3 tablespoons		
Bread Sticks	4-9″ long		
Tortillas	1-6″ diameter		

Cereals | Amount

Cereals	Amount
All Bran	½ cup
Bran Flakes	½ cup
Other ready to eat unsweetened cereal	¾ cup
Puffed cereal (unsweetened)	1 cup
Cereal, cooked	½ cup
Grits, cooked	½ cup
Rice, cooked	½ cup
Barley, cooked	½ cup
Pasta, cooked (noodle products)	½ cup
Popcorn (popped without fat)	3 cups
Cornmeal	2 tablespoons
Flour	2 ½ tablespoons
Wheat germ	¼ cup
Cornstarch	2 tablespoons

Miscellaneous Foods | Amount

Miscellaneous Foods	Amount
Ice Cream (omit 2 fat exchanges)	½ cup
French Fries (omit 1 fat exchange)	8 3″ × ½″
Potato Chips (omit 2 fat exchanges)	15
Corn Chips (omit 2 fat exchanges)	15

Starchy Vegetables	Amount
Beans (dried and cooked)	1/2 cup
Peas (dried and cooked)	1/2 cup
Lentils (dried and cooked)	1/2 cup
Peas (green canned or frozen)	1/2 cup
Corn (canned or frozen)	1/3 cup
Corn on the cob	1 small
Lima beans	1/2 cup
Parsnips	2/3 cup
Potato (white)	1 small
Potato, mashed	1/2 cup
Potato (sweet)	1/4 cup
Pumpkin	3/4 cup
Squash (winter)	1/2 cup
Yam	1/4 cup

• Starchy vegetables are included in the bread exchange list as they contain the same amount of protein and carbohydrate as one slice of bread.

LIST 5: MEAT EXCHANGES

Meat is divided into three categories. Each LEAN MEAT EXCHANGE contains 7 grams of protein, 3 grams of fat and 55 calories. For each MEDIUM-FAT MEAT EXCHANGE count 75 calories and omit 1/2 fat exchange. For each HIGH-FAT MEAT EXCHANGE count 100 calories and omit 1 fat exchange.

	Low-Fat Meat Exchanges	Amount
(Fat Removed)		
Beef:	Baby beef, chopped beef, chuck, flank steak, london broil, tenderloin plate, ribs, top and bottom round (steak and roast), all cuts rump, sirloin and tripe	1 ounce
Lamb:	Leg, rib, loin, shoulder and shank	1 ounce
Pork:	Leg, rump, center shank, smoked ham (center slices)	1 ounce
Veal:	Leg, loin, rib, cutlets	1 ounce
Poultry:	Flesh only (skin removed), chicken, turkey, Cornish game hen, pheasant	1 ounce

Seafoods		
and Fish:	Any fresh or frozen fish	1 ounce
	Canned salmon, tuna, mackerel, crab or lobster	1/4 cup
	Clams, oysters, scallops, shrimp	1 ounce or 5 medium
	Sardines, drained	3
Cheese:	Those containing less than 5% butterfat	1 ounce

<u>Low-Fat Meat Exchange</u>	<u>Amount</u>
Cottage Cheese: Dry, 2% butterfat	$1/4$ cup

• Check pre-basted and liquid cured meats and poultry for sugar and fat contents.

<u>Medium-Fat Meat Exchanges</u>

Beef: Ground (15% fat) corned beef (canned), rib eye, ground round	1 ounce
Pork: Loin (all cuts), shoulder (picnic), Boston butt, broiled ham, Canadian bacon	1 ounce
All: Liver, heart, kidney, sweetbreads	1 ounce
Cheese: Mozzarella, Ricotta, Farmer's Cheese,	1 ounce
Parmesan, grated	3 tablespoons
Eggs: Raw or cooked (no fat added)	1

High-Fat Meat Exchanges

	Amount
Beef: Ground beef (more than 20% fat), corned beef brisket, brisket, commercial hamburger, chuck, rib roasts and steaks	1 ounce
Veal: Breast	1 ounce
Lamb: Breast	1 ounce
Pork: Spare ribs, loin, ground pork, sausage, country style ham, deviled ham	1 ounce
Poultry: Duck, goose	1 ounce
Cheese: Cheddar	1 ounce
Prepared	
Meats: Frankfurters, weiners	1 small
Cold cuts ($4^{1}/_{2}''$ × $^{1}/_{8}''$ slice)	1

LIST 6: FAT EXCHANGES

Each fat exchange contains 5 grams of fat and 45 calories.

Saturated Fats	Amounts
Margarine (regular)	1 teaspoon
Butter	1 teaspoon
Bacon Grease	1 teaspoon
Bacon, cooked crisp	1 slice
Cream, light	2 tablespoons
Cream, sour	2 tablespoons
Cream, heavy	1 tablespoon
Cream cheese	1 tablespoon
Mayonnaise	1 teaspoon
Salad dressing (mayonnaise type)	2 teaspoons
Lard	1 teaspoon

Polyunsaturated Fats	
Soft margarine (tub or stick)	1 teaspoon
Avocado	$1/8$-4″ diameter
Corn Oil	1 teaspoon

Polyunsaturated Fats	Amounts
Cottonseed Oil	1 teaspoon
Safflower Oil	1 teaspoon
Soy Oil	1 teaspoon
Sunflower Oil	1 teaspoon
Olive Oil	1 teaspoon
Peanut Oil	1 teaspoon
Olives	5 small
Nuts:	
Almonds	10 whole
Pecans	2 large
Spanish Peanuts	20 whole
Virginia Peanuts	10 whole
Walnuts	6 small
Other Nuts	6 small

Fats are concentrated calorie sources and should be measured carefully. The origin of fat is either animal or vegetable and they range from solid hard fats to liquid oils. Generally, vegetable fats (corn oil, peanut oil, etc.) remain liquid at room temperature. Saturated fat is often hard at room temperature and is primarily from animal food products (butter, bacon, meat fat, etc.).

ARTIFICIAL SWEETENERS
NON-CALORIC

Artificial sweeteners are available on the retail market in liquid, powder, tablets, cubes and granules. They replace sugar in sweetening power only and have no calories or food value.

Artificial sweetening agents do not provide the same bulk, texture or preservative quality of sugar. Please refrigerate artificially sweetened foods for safe keeping. This will reduce spoilage.

When cooking with artificial sweeteners, be wary of their peculiarities. Undissolved powder or tablets will taste excessively sweet. To avoid this, simply crush and/or dissolve sweeteners in a bit of the liquid in a recipe, or mix in a small amount of water to use as desired. Tablets dissolve fastest in warm water.

Saccharin may give off a bitter flavor, especially after heating. To avoid this aftertaste, simply sweeten as near to the end of cooking as possible, and only use the smallest amount necessary.

Products differ and experimenting will help you decide which textures, types and flavors you prefer. Equivalents are given on the labels and vary from product to product. Each time you buy a product check the label for changes in the sugar equivalent. As products are improved, the equivalent amounts often change.

Too much artificial sweetener often leaves a bitter tang, usually a little salt will counteract this objectionable taste. Be careful not to over salt. Too much salt can also ruin your product.

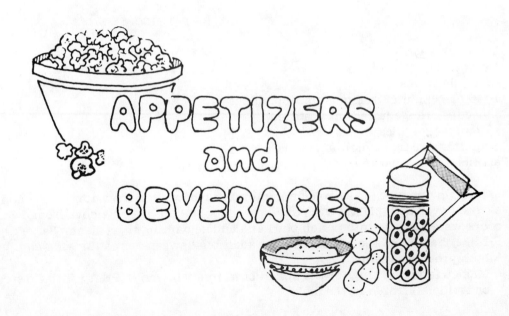

APPETIZERS
and
BEVERAGES

SPICY FRUIT PUNCH

Makes 24 servings
1/2 cup serving equals
1/2 fruit exchange
20 calories
C-5   P-0   F-0

1 1/2 cups water
1 cinnamon stick
12 whole cloves
1 (46 oz.) can unsweetened pineapple juice
1 1/2 cups orange juice (unsweetened)
1/2 cup lemon juice
1 quart sugar free lemon-lime soda
artificial sweetener to equal 1/4 cup sugar if desired

In a one quart casserole or small mixing bowl mix the water, cinnamon and cloves. Cover with plastic wrap and bring to a boil on high. Remove from oven and let cool covered. Strain into punch bowl and add remaining ingredients. Serve over ice.
- I like the tang of the punch without additional sweetener as the soda and juices both provide sweetness.
- Make a fancy ice ring for the punch bowl in a jello mold. Pretty with flowers (fresh or artificial) frozen in the mold.

HOT CHOCOLATE

4 servings
1 serving equals
1 skim milk exchange
80 calories
C-12 P-8 F-1

3 tablespoons cocoa
3 cups skim milk
artificial sweetener to equal 1 tablespoon sugar

Place cocoa and milk in glass 1 quart measuring cup. Heat 3-4 minutes on high until hot but not boiling. Stir twice while heating. Remove from micro and let set 2 minutes before adding sweetener. Pour into individual mugs.

MOCK TOM & JERRY

1 cup skim milk
artificial sweetener to taste
dash of cinnamon or nutmeg
rum or brandy extract to taste

1 cup equals
1 skim milk exchange
80 calories
C-12 P-8 F-0

Heat milk on high one minute. Stir and add flavoring to taste and heat an additional 15-20 seconds. Take care not to boil milk. Let rest 1-2 minutes and add sweetener. Sprinkle with your favorite spice.

WINTER WARMER

Serves 4
1 serving equals
$3/4$ fruit exchange
30 calories
C-8   P-0   F-0

3 cups low calorie cran-apple juice
8 whole cloves
4 broken cinnamon sticks

    Combine all ingredients in 1 quart measuring cup. Heat on high 2–3 minutes. Reduce heat to medium low (40%) power and cook 7–8 minutes. Strain into mugs. Wait 3–4 minutes before drinking.
    Good on cold winter nights, for Halloween parties or after a snowy day.
• This is really pretty served in a carafe on a buffet table—and it smells inviting too.

HOT DOG MAN

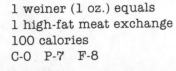

1 weiner (1 oz.) equals
1 high-fat meat exchange
100 calories
C-0   P-7   F-8

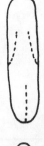

Slit weiner as indicated by dotted lines. Micro on high on a paper plate for 1 minute. As weiner cooks, arms will curl outward and legs will spread apart. Give him a face, buttons, and tie his shoes with the mustard squeezer.

These are a real delight at youth groups and kiddy parties—not to mention a rainy day lunch!

QUICK ZIPPY CHEESE DIP

Makes 1 cup
8 servings
2 tablespoons equal
75 calories
1 medium-fat meat exchange
C-0   P-7   F-5.5

8 ounces processed cheese
1 tablespoon jalapeno relish

Cut cheese into small cubes and place in small glass casserole. Cook on medium high (80%) 1 minute. Stir in the relish and cook an additional minute. Stir and cover with waxed paper 2–3 minutes to carryover cook and continue melting the cheese. If cheese is not completely melted cook an additional minute. For a thinner dip add 1 tablespoon skim milk with the relish. Let rest 5 minutes before serving. Serve warm.
• This is most enjoyable with vegetable sticks, tortilla chips or crusty bread cubes.
• Makes a dip with a Mexican flavor flair that is rather colorful with the green peppery flecks.
• For a spicy dip increase the jalapeno relish—add small amounts at a time as relish is powerful!

DEVILED CRAB/SHRIMP DIP

32 servings
1 tablespoon equals
50 calories
$1/2$ low-fat meat exchange
$1/2$ fat exchange
C-0   P-4   F-4

1 (8 oz.) package cream cheese
1 cup crab, shrimp or a combination
2 tablespoons chopped sweet onion
2 tablespoons skim milk
$1/2$ teaspoon horseradish
$1/2$ teaspoon salt
$1/2$ teaspoon pepper
$1/4$ teaspoon dry mustard

Soften cream cheese in micro on high 2 minutes unwrapped in a glass dish. Mix all remaining ingredients into cheese and bake on medium high for 4–6 minutes or until hot.

Serve with vegetable sticks, French bread cubes or crackers. Vegetable sticks are free.

CRAB & CHEESE BITES

36 appetizers
1 appetizer equals
1/4 low-fat meat exchange
1/2 fat exchange
1/5 bread exchange
55 calories
C-3   P-3   F-3

8 ounces crab meat
1 teaspoon sliced green onion
4 ounces shredded Swiss cheese
1/4 cup mayonnaise
1 teaspoon lemon juice
1/4 teaspoon curry powder
1/8 teaspoon pepper
36 melba toast rounds

Combine first seven ingredients and mix well. Spoon crab mixture on toast rounds. Place half of rounds on a microwave baking tray lined with paper towels. Heat on 70% power 20-30 seconds or until mixture is warm and cheese is melted. Repeat with other half of appetizers. These are good on the onion or sesame melba rounds.

TUNA SNACKERS

36 appetizers
1 appetizer equals
$1/4$ low-fat meat exchange
$1/2$ fat exchange
$1/6$ bread exchange
55 calories
C-3   P-3   F-3

8 ounces tuna fish packed in water (drained)
1 teaspoon sliced green onion
4 ounces shredded Swiss or
   American cheese
$1/4$ cup mayonnaise
1 teaspoon lemon juice
1 teaspoon chopped pimento
$1/8$ teaspoon pepper
36 rye melba toast rounds

     Combine first seven ingredients and mix well. Spoon tuna mixture on rye rounds. Place half of rounds on micro baking dish lined with paper towels. Heat on 80% power approximately 25 seconds until mixture is warm and cheese melted.
• Use rye toast cut into strips (5 per slice) in place of melba toast if desired.
• The paper towel keeps the crackers or toast crispy.

CHEESE EMPANADAS

1 turnover equals
1/2 high-fat meat exchange
1 bread exchange
C-15   P-6   F-4
120 calories
1 strip equals
20 calories
C-3   P-1   F-1

1 corn tortilla or flour tortilla
1/2 slice or 2 tablespoons shredded cheddar or Jack cheese

Heat tortilla on a paper towel for 30 seconds on high. Place cheese on one half and fold over (turnover style) to cover cheese. Heat an additional 20–30 seconds for cheese to melt. Cut into six strips and nibble away.
• Great as an appetizer or a nice change from a sandwich with soup or a salad.
• The micro softens the tortilla without frying in fat!

COCKTAIL CHICKEN WINGS

About 30 pieces
1 piece equals
$1/4$ low-fat meat exchange
15 calories
C-0   P-2   F-1

14–15 chicken wings (approximately 3 pounds)
$1/2$ cup salad oil
$1/2$ cup lemon juice
1 clove garlic, quartered
1 teaspoon salt
$1/2$ teaspoon pepper
$1/4$ teaspoon paprika

Cut wings apart at both joints and discard tips. Often your butcher will cut chicken wings apart at no additional charge. Marinate chicken parts in remaining ingredients at least an hour. Cover chicken with wax paper and cook on high for 6 minutes. Turn chicken over and continue as above for about 6 more minutes. Chicken should be tender, not hard and dry. Let rest 5 minutes before serving. Serve with napkins.
• If wings look small check for doneness a bit early.

YE OLDE SNACKIN' CEREAL

Serves 8
1 serving (scant half cup)
equals
1/2 bread exchange
1/2 fat exchange
60 calories
C-8   P-1   F-2.5

2¼ cups Rice or Corn Chex
1 cup Wheat Chex
½ cup thin pretzel sticks
4 teaspoons butter or margarine
2 teaspoons Worcestershire sauce
½ teaspoon garlic salt

Melt butter or margarine in custard cup on high 30 seconds. Add Worcestershire sauce and garlic salt and heat an additional 15 seconds. Mix well. Drizzle butter sauce over cereal mix in a flat glass baking dish. Cook on medium high (80%) 3–4 minutes, stirring every minute (or the cereal will burn on the bottom). Cool and store in a covered container.
• I usually make mix in a deep dish 10 inch pie plate as it has lots of stirring room.
• Good nibble in lunches or for card and party snacks.

CRISPY TORTILLA CHIPS

16 pieces equals
1 bread exchange
70 calories
C-15   P-2   F-0

corn tortillas (the kind from the grocer's
   refrigerated case)

   Cut tortilla into 16 pie shaped wedges and place on a paper towel. Micro high $1^1/_2$–$2^1/_2$ minutes uncovered. Remove from oven and let cool. Tortilla bits will be crispy when cool. Do not let brown.
   Presto! Fat-free chips to nibble or dip.
• Time varies by temperature and thickness of tortilla.
• These are also good sprinkled with your favorite seasonings and/or salt.

SMOKEY JERKY

Serves 8
1 serving equals
1 low-fat meat exchange
55 calories
C-0   P-7   F-3

$1^1/_2$–2 pounds lean boneless beef (flank, brisket or round—lean only)
$^1/_4$ cup soy sauce
1 tablespoon Worcestershire sauce
$^1/_4$ teaspoons pepper, garlic powder, onion powder
$^3/_4$ teaspoon hickory smoke flavored salt OR increase garlic powder to $^1/_2$ teaspoon

Partially freeze the meat before slicing to make it easier to slice evenly. Cut the meat with the grain of the beef if you prefer chewy jerky and across the grain for a more tender, but brittle jerky. Slice beef $^1/_8$ inch thick and set aside. Mix remaining ingredients and add beef strips. Marinate an hour at room temperature. Micro high, covered with a paper towel to catch the splatters, for $2^1/_2$ minutes. Remove towel and turn meat over. Micro another $1^1/_2$–$2^1/_2$ minutes until meat has browned and appears dry. Let cool and finish drying at room temperature. Makes about $^1/_2$ pound.

• If the jerky is completely dried before removing from the microwave it will cool an unbelievable cross between a rock and cardboard. Watch near the end of cooking time as size of strip and temperature will have some effect on time.

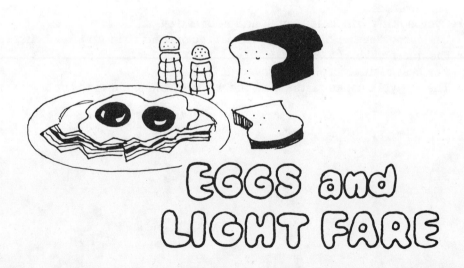

EGGS and LIGHT FARE

EGG TIPS

- For fluffier scrambled eggs, stir the egg mixture frequently.
- To avoid "super mess" take eggs out of the shell before cooking. Eggs in the shell build up a tremendous amount of pressure and are very likely to explode. There's nothing worse than cleaning egg particles out of every corner and the top portion of your oven!
- Eggs poach evenly when completely covered with water.
- Exact cooking time of microwave cooked eggs will vary according to egg size and temperature.
- Overcooking will cause tough and rubbery eggs.
- Undercook eggs a bit as they will carryover and firm up after being removed from the microwave.
- For best results, cook eggs covered.
- The egg yolk cooks faster than the white of the egg due to the higher fat content.

BAKED EGG

1 egg equals
1 medium-fat meat exchange
$1/2$ fat exchange
98 calories
C-0   P-6   F-8

1 egg
$1/2$ teaspoon butter or margarine

Break egg into custard cup that has been greased with the butter or margarine. Microwave low—covered with plastic wrap—for one minute or until egg reaches desired degree of doneness. Uncover and serve hot.

Baked eggs are kind of a cross between poached and fried eggs. I like them on toast or used in eggs Benedict. They are super topped with cheese sauce.

Baked eggs cooked hard are great chopped up for use in salads or any recipe calling for hard cooked eggs.

MICRO McMUFFIN

Serves 2
1 serving equals
1 medium-fat meat exchange
1 low-fat meat exchange
1 high-fat meat exchange
2 bread exchanges
370 calories
C-30   P-24   F-24

2 eggs, baked (page 38)
2 slices Canadian bacon
2 slices American cheese (1 oz. each)
2 whole English muffins, toasted if desired

Bake eggs and keep covered. Toast muffins in toaster while heating bacon in a single layer on a paper towel on high for $1^1/_4$–$1^1/_2$ minutes. When muffins are ready place bacon, egg, and cheese on two muffin halves and top with remaining muffins. Wrap sandwich in a paper towel and heat 1–$1^1/_2$ minutes on medium power (60%).
Breakfast out, in—anytime!

MEATY EGG FOO YUNG
(nice light meal)

Serves 4
1 serving equals
$1/2$ fat exchange
1 medium-fat meat exchange
$1/2$ vegetable exchange
1 low-fat meat exchange
165 calories
C-5   P-10   F-10

2 teaspoons butter or margarine
4 eggs
$1/2$ pound fresh bean sprouts
4–5 sliced green onions (tops too)
1 cup cooked small shrimp, crab or cut up cooked chicken or pork
$1/4$ teaspoon salt
$1/8$ teaspoon pepper
$1/8$ teaspoon granulated garlic powder

Wash and drain bean sprouts and set aside. Melt butter in a 9 inch glass pie pan. Beat eggs and add remaining ingredients. Add to butter and cook uncovered 5 minutes on high stirring cooked portion toward center each minute so liquid can flow to sides and bottom of dish. Cut into wedges and serve with soy sauce or any leftover fat-free gravy if chicken or pork is used.

HANGTOWN FRY

Serves 1
equals
1 fat exchange
2 medium-fat meat exchanges
1 low-fat meat exchange
250 calories
C-0   P-21   F-20

1 slice diced bacon
1/4 cup chopped oysters (approximately 3 small or 2 medium)
2 eggs
1 teaspoon water
1/4 teaspoon Worcestershire sauce, if desired for zip
salt and pepper to taste

Place bacon in a 9 inch glass pie plate, cover with platic wrap and cook on high 1 minute. Add oysters, cover and cook on high an additional minute. While bacon and oysters are cooking, beat remaining ingredients together. Stir egg mixture into oysters, cover and cook—stirring 3 times—about 1 1/2 minutes or until eggs are set to your liking. These will carryover cook slightly after being removed from the oven.

WESTERN EGG

Serves 1
equals
2 medium-fat meat exchanges
$^1/_2$ fat exchange
vegetable exchange negligible
175 calories
C-0 P-15 F-9

$^1/_2$ teaspoon butter or margarine
$^1/_4$ cup diced cooked ham
$^1/_2$ teaspoon chopped onion
1 teaspoon chopped green pepper
1 egg

    Melt butter in an 8 inch glass pie plate. Mix remaining ingredients and pour into pie pan. Cover and cook on medium high (80%) for 1 minute. Stir carefully. Cook an additional 30 seconds or until set.

WESTERN EGG SANDWICH

Serves 1
one sandwich equals
2 medium-fat meat exchanges
$1/2$ fat exchange
2 bread exchanges
vegetable exchange negligible
315 calories
C-30   P-19   F-9

$1/2$ teaspoon butter or margarine
$1/4$ cup diced cooked ham
$1/2$ teaspoon chopped green pepper
1 egg
2 slices bread, toasted or one hamburger bun

Melt butter in an 8 inch glass pie plate. Mix remaining ingredients and pour into pie pan. Cover and cook on medium high (80%) for 1 minute. Stir carefully. Cook an additional 30 seconds until set. Place egg between two slices of toast or on the bun. Wrap in a paper towel and micro 15–20 seconds to heat through.

This is a good warm sandwich for breakfast, lunch or brunch.

BASIC OMELETTE

One basic omelette
equals
1 fat exchange
2 medium-fat meat exchanges
195 calories
C-0   P-12   F-16

2 eggs
2 tablespoons water or skim milk
¼ teaspoon salt
dash of pepper
1 teaspoon butter or margarine

Place butter in glass pie plate and melt on high 30 seconds. In a small bowl beat the eggs, water, salt and pepper until light and frothy. Tilt butter plate to coat bottom of dish and a bit on the sides. Pour in egg mixture and cover with plastic wrap. Micro 1½ minutes on simmer/defrost (30%). Pull cooked portion along edges toward center with spatula so uncooked portions flow to the outside. Cover again and continue cooking 1¼–1½ minutes. While top is moist and creamy looking place desired filling on one half. With spatula fold omelette in half over filling or roll up. Let the omelette rest covered about a minute for the internal heat to warm the filling.

Serve hot and enjoy.

• I generally add filling and make 2 servings at breakfast.

Omelettes are nourishing entrees for any meal. At lunch I often have one with a tossed salad and if served for a light dinner I accompany it with a vegetable, fruit cup and muffin.

These are great "in a hurry" meals that even make use of leftover bits of meat, cheeses and vegetables.

OMELETTE VARIATIONS

• Ingredients other than basic omelette recipe are fillings.

DENVER OMELETTE

1 basic omelette recipe
1/4 cup cooked diced ham
1 tablespoon diced green onion
1 teaspoon chopped onion (or a thin slice with the rings separated)

Whole Omelette	2 servings
equals	equals
1 low-fat meat exchange	1/2 low-fat meat exchange
2 medium-fat meat exchanges	1 medium-fat meat exchange
1 fat exchange	1/2 fat exchange
vegetable exchange negligible	vegetable exchange negligible
250 calories	125 calories
C-0 P-21 P-19	C-0 P-10 F-10

SEAFOOD AND CHEESE OMELETTE

1 basic omelette recipe
1/4 cup crab, shrimp or a combination
1/4 cup grated cheddar or Swiss cheese or 1 (1 oz.) slice American

Whole Omelette
equals
1 low-fat meat exchange
1 high-fat meat exchange
2 medium-fat meat exchanges
1 fat exchange
350 calories
C-0 P-29 F-29

2 servings
equals
1/2 low-fat meat exchange
1/2 high-fat meat exchange
1 medium-fat meat exchange
1/2 fat exchange
175 calories
C-0 P-15 F-14

- For a Ham and Cheese omelette, substitute ham for the seafood and the exchanges and calories remain the same.
- For a Ham omelette just add ham and deduct 1 high-fat meat exchange and 100 calories from the whole omelette above. When you omit the cheese the CPF values for the whole omelette are C-0 P-22 F-21.

OMELETTE SUPREME

1 basic omelette recipe
1/4 cup cooked chicken or turkey bits
1/4 cup grated cheddar or Swiss cheese
2 tablespoons mushrooms, drained (if fresh mushrooms are used, slice and cook covered about 20 seconds on high heat in the butter. Remove from butter—set aside 100and proceed as usual.)

Whole Omelette	2 servings
equals	equals
2 medium-fat meat exchanges	1 medium-fat meat exchange
1 fat exchange	1/2 fat exchange
1 high-fat meat exchange	1/2 high-fat meat exchange
1 low-fat meat exchange	1/2 low-fat meat exchange
1/4 vegetable exchange	vegetable exchange negligible
355 calories	175 calories
C-0 P-29 F-29	C-0 P-15 F-14

- This makes a nice light meal after the "holiday food" assortment and uses up leftover bits of the turkey!
- Fresh mushrooms make a richer omelette.

CHEESE OMELETTE

1 basic omelette recipe
1/4 cup grated cheddar or Swiss cheese or 1 (1 oz.) slice American

Whole Omelette
equals
1 high-fat meat exchange
2 medium-fat meat exchanges
1 fat exchange
295 calories
C-0   P-20   F-26

2 servings
equals
1/2 high-fat meat exchange
1 medium-fat meat exchange
1/2 fat exchange
148 calories
C-0   P-10   F-13

- I like American cheese with pimento for a change (1 teaspoon).
- A tablespoon of cooked mushrooms is also good with cheese for filling.
- Pimento or mushroom exchanges are negligible in these amounts.

SUNDAY MORNING QUICHE

Serves 6
1 serving equals (filling only)
1 medium-fat meat exchange
1 high-fat meat exchange
$1/3$ milk exchange
205 calories
C-4   P-17   F-13.5
Shell adds the following
per serving (6 servings)
1 bread exchange
2 fat exchanges
160 calories
C-15   P-2   F-10
(recipe on page 148)

1 baked 9″ pie shell
3 large eggs
$2/3$ cup evaporated milk (1 small 5.33 oz. can)
1 tablespoon finely minced onion or 1 green onion chopped
$1/4$ cup sliced fresh mushrooms
$3/4$ cup chopped cooked ham, crab, or shrimp
1 tablespoon chopped green pepper or celery, if desired
1 cup grated cheese cheddar, Swiss or a combination

Mix eggs, grated cheese and milk—set aside. In bottom of the baked pie shell combine onion, mushrooms, ham and green pepper or celery. Pour egg mixture over filling. Cook uncovered on medium high (80%) for 4 minutes. Turn quiche 1/4 turn and continue cooking 4 more minutes. Center will still jiggle slightly. Cover with waxed paper and rest 2 minutes. If center is too soft for your liking cover outer edges of filling with foil and cook another 30–45 seconds. Center holds heat—wait 3–4 minutes before serving.

• To help set the center and keep edges cooking evenly, I often stir the filling when I rotate the dish. Take care when doing this not to poke holes in the bottom of the crust.
• For better cooking action underneath, bake the quiche on your bacon rack.
• If cooked on high power, the edges will dry out and toughen before the center of the pie is cooked.

CREAMED TUNA
(no fats added)

Serves 3
1 serving equals
$1/4$ bread exchange
$1/2$ milk exchange
$1^1/2$ low-fat meat exchanges
140 calories
C-11   P-18   F-6
On toast add (per slice)
1 bread exchange
70 calories
C-15   P-2   F-0

$1^1/2$ cups skim milk
2 tablespoons flour
$1/2$ teaspoon salt
$1/4$ teaspoon pepper
1 (6 oz.) can water-packed tuna fish

Drain tuna and set aside. Heat milk in a 1 quart casserole on high about 20 seconds. Mix the flour in a small amount of cold water to form a smooth paste. Stir into milk with a wire whip. (Don't leave whip in the microwave.) Cook on high, stirring every 30 seconds until mixture is smooth and thickened. Remove from microwave

50

and flake in tuna. Heat covered with waxed paper 1 minute. Keep covered with the waxed paper and let rest 3–4 minutes before serving.

- Great hot lunch served on toast!
- My dad likes cooked frozen peas sprinkled on his creamed tuna. If you do add the peas—remember to add the exchanges and calories.
- Substitute cooked chicken or turkey for the tuna for great la king meals and serve on a biscuit instead of toast. This makes leftovers into a plan over. A teaspoon of chopped pimento is good with the chicken or turkey and will not change the values. Calculations are the same with the chicken or turkey as with tuna fish.

DELUXE CREAMED CHIPPED BEEF

Serves 4
1 serving equals
$1/3$ bread exchange
$1/2$ milk exchange
$1/2$ high-fat meat exchange
1 low-fat meat exchange
vegetable exchange negligible
(if mushrooms are added)
170 calories
C-15 P-18 F-7

2 cups skim milk
4 tablespoons flour
$1/3$ cup water
$1/4$ teaspoon pepper
$1/2$ cup grated cheddar cheese (medium or sharp)
$1/4$ cup drained mushrooms, if desired
1 small jar dried beef

- I like to place beef in strainer and blanche with boiling water to remove excess salt and let it drain while cooking the sauce. Check your beef for salt—not all brands are excessively salty but many would ruin your entree if not blanched. Packaged beef is usually not as salty as that in the jar.

    Heat milk on high in a 2 quart casserole for about 45 seconds. Mix the flour in the water to form a smooth paste. Stir flour mixture into milk with wire whip and cook on high, stirring each 30 seconds until mixture is thickened and bubbly. Stir in cheese and mushrooms and cook covered with waxed paper $1–1 1/4$ minutes. Remove from microwave and stir in drained beef. Cover tightly and let rest 5 minutes to finish melting the cheese and heat the beef, letting the flavors blend.

- This is yummy on toast or biscuits and makes a super brunch treat or a nice light luncheon or dinner.
- If serving on toast or biscuit add (per slice or biscuit) 1 bread exchange, 70 calories and C-15   P-2   F-0.

BACON

1 slice equals
1 fat exchange
45 calories
C-0   P-0   F-5

Arrange bacon on a bacon rack or paper plate (paper plate is good only for 1–2 pieces or grease will flow in bottom of oven) and cover with a paper towel. The towel prevents splattering and absorbs much grease. Cook as follows on high power:

1–2 slices	1–1$^1/_2$ minutes
3 slices	1$^1/_2$–2 minutes
4 slices	2–3 minutes
8 slices	4–5$^1/_2$ minutes

Remove from oven and let bacon stand 1 minute to crisp.
• The cooking time varies on bacon because of the thickness, temperature, curing process and degree of doneness preferred. Be sure to check at the earliest time and go from there. Different brands cook in different amounts of time.

53

SKINNY TUNA ASPIC

1 package (tablespoon)
  unflavored gelatine
1³/₄ cups tomato juice
1 teaspoon Worcestershire sauce
2 tablespoons lemon juice
¹/₄ teaspoon salt
1 can (6 oz.) tuna fish, drained
³/₄ cup finely chopped celery
1 tablespoon finely chopped
  green onion

Serves 8
1 serving equals
¹/₂ vegetable exchange
¹/₂ low-fat meat exchange
40 calories
C-2.5 P-4.5 F-1.5
Serves 4
1 vegetable exchange
1 low-fat meat exchange
80 calories
C-5 P-9 F-3

Soften gelatine in 1 cup tomato juice about 2 minutes in a one quart glass bowl. Micro on high 2 minutes stirring once. Add remaining tomato juice, Worcestershire sauce, lemon juice and salt. Mix well and refrigerate until mixture begins to thicken. Add flaked drained tuna, celery and green onion. Fold gently into thickened mixture. Pour into mold and refrigerate until set. Serves 8 if used as part of a meal or on a buffet, etc., or serves 4 if put into individual molds.
• Good hot day lunch and simple to prepare.
• A bit of chopped green pepper may be added if desired.

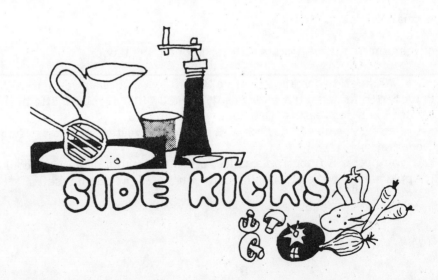

SIDE KICKS

QUICK APPLE SAUCE

Serves 4
1 serving equals
1 fruit exchange
40 calories
C-10   P-0   F-0

4 small apples, peeled
1/3 cup water
cinnamon or nutmeg to taste (I use about 1/2 teaspoon)

Wash and slice apples into a 2 quart glass casserole dish. Add water and cover. Cook 5–7 minutes until fruit is soft cooked but not mush. Stir in seasonings. Let rest 5 minutes before eating. Delicious warm or cold.
• If a sweeter sauce is desired add artificial sweetener to taste after cooking and cooling.
• If you prefer a finer apple sauce, press through a sieve after cooking.
• Apple sauce is the all-time favorite with pork at our house.

CREOLE SAUCE

Makes 1 cup
$1/4$ cup equals
$1/4$ bread exchange
$1/2$ fat exchange
vegetable exchange negligible
40 calories
C-4   P-.5   F-2.5

2 tablespoons chopped green pepper
2 tablespoons chopped onion
2 tablespoons chopped celery, if desired
2 teaspoons butter or margarine
$1/8$ teaspoon garlic powder
$1/4$ teaspoon chili powder
1 can (8 oz.) tomato sauce

In a 1 quart casserole heat the first four ingredients covered on high $2^{1}/_{2}$ minutes. Add remaining ingredients, stir and cook covered 3–4 minutes, stirring once. Let sauce rest covered 5 minutes before serving.
• Great with fish. Can be placed on raw fish and the flavors will cook through.
• Makes a super omelette topping and is good with leftover chicken or seafood pieces on rice.
• I also like the sauce on green cooked veggies like zucchini.

WHITE SAUCE

Thin	Medium	Thick
1 cup skim milk	1 cup skim milk	1 cup skim milk
1 tablespoon flour	2 tablespoons flour	3 tablespoons flour
1 tablespoon water	2 tablespoons water	3 tablespoons water
1 cup equals	1 cup equals	1 cup equals
1 milk exchange	1 milk exchange	1 milk exchange
1/3 bread exchange	2/3 bread exchange	1 bread exchange
105 calories	130 calories	150 calories
C-17 P-9 F-0	C-22 P-9 F-0	C-27 P-10 F-0

Heat milk 20–25 seconds on high. Mix flour with cold water to form smooth paste. Mix in milk and stir well with wire whip. Cook on high about four minutes, stirring every 30 seconds until smooth and thick. Stirring is a must or thickener will cook on the bottom of the dish. Remove from oven and allow to rest 3–4 minutes before serving. Season with salt and pepper to taste.

• A hint of onion powder gives a bit of zip to white sauce.

CHEESE SAUCE

Makes 1 cup
1/2 cup equals
1/3 bread exchange
1/2 milk exchange
1/2 high-fat meat exchange
115 calories
C-11   P-9   F-4

1 cup skim milk
2 tablespoons flour
1/2 teaspoon salt
1/4 teaspoon pepper
1/4 cup grated or 1 ounce diced sharp cheddar cheese

Heat milk on high about 15 seconds. Mix flour with a small amount of cold water to make a smooth paste and stir paste into milk with wire whip. Cook on high stirring every 30 seconds until mixture is smooth and thickened. Stirring is important to keep thickener mixed with milk or it will cook on the bottom of your container. Stir in cheese and cook 1 additional minute. Cover and let rest 3–4 minutes to carryover cook and finish melting the cheese. Do not micro on high until cheese is completely melted as it may curdle.

Excellent over vegetables or open-faced hot sandwiches.

QUICK CHEESE SAUCE

Serves 4
1 serving equals
1 high-fat meat exchange
milk exchange negligible
100 calories
C-0   P-7   F-8

¼ cup skim milk
½ cup grated processed cheese (Velveeta type)
   or 4 ounces cubed
dash of dry mustard

Mix milk, cheese and dash of dry mustard. Cover with waxed paper and cook on high 2 minutes, stirring half way through cooking. Remove from micro and let rest covered 2–3 minutes for cheese to finish melting. Stir twice during carryover time.

Good on vegetables or open-faced sandwiches.
• Kids like this used as a fondue with crusty French bread and cooked meat cubes.

JELLIED CRANBERRY SAUCE

Serves 10–12
Free food
Calories and exchanges
are negligible

4 cups fresh cranberries
$1^1/_4$ cup water
1 envelope unflavored gelatine dissolved in $^1/_4$ cup cold water
artificial sweetener to equal $^3/_4$ cup sugar

 In a 3 quart casserole combine water and washed cranberries. Cook on high 7–8 minutes until berries pop and mixture boils. Stir 4 times during cooking. Remove from micro and stir in the gelatine mixture. Continue stirring until gelatine is completely mixed and dissolved. Cover tightly and let carryover cook for 10 minutes, stirring after 6 minutes and adding sweetener. Chill in casserole or salad mold.
• The gelatine prevents the artificially sweetened berries from being watery. In sugar-sweetened cranberries the sugar gets syrupy and helps thicken the sauce.

BAKED POTATOES

1 small potato
equals
1 bread exchange
70 calories
C-15   P-2   F-0

Scrub potatoes and clip off ends. Prick sides of potatoes with sharp knife or fork about $1/2$ inch deep in four places. This allows the steam to escape and helps avoid an exploded potato and super mess. I can't imagine a worse mess than cleaning potato out of the little vent holes!

Bake on rack or paper towel according to the following chart, turning the potatoes over half way through cooking time. Let rest (covered with a dish towel) 10 minutes to carryover cook and avoid burning the diner. Check for fork tenderness. Potatoes will remain warm a good half hour.

1 potato	3–5 minutes	3 potatoes	7–10 minutes
2 potatoes	5–7 minutes	4 potatoes	10–12 minutes

• One half slice cheese ($1/2$ oz.) and a sprinkling of dried chives tucked in a small slit during carryover time is a nice added touch for a change. Add $1/2$ high-fat meat, 50 calories and C-0   P-3.5   F-4.

STUFFED POTATOES

Serves 4
1 serving equals
1 bread exchange
$1/4$ high-fat meat exchange
milk exchange negligible
100 calories
C-15 P-4 F-2

2 large potatoes
$1/2$ teaspoon onion powder
2 tablespoons skim milk
$1/4$ cup grated cheddar cheese
salt and pepper to taste
paprika for garnish

Scrub and pierce potatoes with knife about 4 times and cut off ends. Bake on high 6 minutes, turning after 3. Let cool, covered, about 15 minutes. Cut in half lengthwise and carefully scoop out centers leaving shells intact. Mash centers with onion powder, milk, salt and pepper. Stir in grated cheese. Refill shells ($1/4$ of the mixture each) and sprinkle tops with paprika. Heat on high about $1^{1}/_{4}$ minutes until warm through.
- Great do-ahead for busy days or company meals. Do ahead, refrigerate and heat adding a bit of extra time (about 2 additional minutes) covered.
- May even be frozen.

SCALLOPED POTATOES

Serves 4
1 serving equals
$1/4$ milk exchange
1 bread exchange
90 calories
C-18   P-4   F-0

2 cups potatotes peeled and sliced (4 small)
1 cup skim milk
salt and pepper to taste
1 tablespoon flour
paprika to garnish

Layer potatoes, flour, salt and pepper in a 2 quart casserole. Pour milk over potatoes and cover. Micro high 14–16 minutes rotating the dish half way through cooking time. Let carryover cook covered 5 minutes. Sprinkle with paprika.
- Larger dish may be used to prevent any chance of bubble-over. Potatoes do cook up sides of dish.
- A sprinkling of onion powder gives the scalloped potatoes a nice flavor.

QUICK MASHED POTATOES

4 small potatoes
1/4 cup milk
1 teaspoon butter or margarine
salt and pepper to taste

Serves 4
1 serving equals
1 bread exchange
1/4 fat exchange
milk negligible
85 calories
C-16   P-2   F-2

Wash and pierce potatoes in 4 places and cut off ends. Place potatoes on a paper towel. Micro high 10–11 minutes turning over half way through cooking time. Let the potatoes rest 5 minutes covered. Peel potatoes and mash adding milk, butter, salt and pepper to taste. Potatoes must be mashed while hot for best results.

FREE GRAVY

1 tablespoon flour or cornstarch
1 cup fat-free drippings or broth
2 drops Kitchen Bouquet for brown gravy or yellow food coloring for light gravy

1/2 cup is a Free food

In a 2 cup glass measuring cup mix liquid and thickener until smooth. Micro high 2–3 minutes until mixture boils and thickens, stirring every minute. Season to taste with salt, pepper or a dash of onion powder, if desired. Micro an additional minute, stirring twice.

SUPER SPUDS

3½ cups frozen southern style
   hash brown potatoes
4 teaspoon dry chopped or
   minced onion
1 cup grated cheddar cheese
1 cup sour cream
1 teaspoon salt
¼ teaspoon pepper

Serves 8
1 serving equals
½ high-fat meat exchange
1 bread exchange
1 fat exchange
165 calories
C-15 P-6 F-9

Topping
¼ cup cornflake crumbs
   (¾ c before crushing)

1 teaspoon butter
• Melt butter and mix

    Thaw potatoes in 8 × 8 casserole or baking dish for 5–6 minutes on medium (50%) stirring once. In a small bowl mix remaining ingredients. Bake uncovered on medium power for 5 minutes. Turn ¼ turn. Cover with waxed paper and micro on medium an additional 9–10 minutes or until heated through and bubbly around the edges. Sprinkle on topping and let rest covered 5 minutes to carryover cook and heat the topping. Enjoy!

• These are great for pot-luck dinners or on a buffet table with cold cuts or baked ham.

CRUMB TOPPING

Makes 1 cup
1/4 cup equals
1/2 bread exchange
1 fat exchange
80 calories
C-8 P-2 F-5

1 cup fresh bread crumbs
1/4 teaspoon paprika
1 tablespoon butter or margarine
1 teaspoon grated Parmesan cheese

Put bread in the blender or use grater to make very fine crumbs. (Store crumbs may be used.) Mix in paprika and grated Parmesan. Melt butter in a 2 cup measuring cup on high about 1 minute. Mix well as you stir in the crumbs.

Sprinkle on any dish that you would like a crumb topping after cooking. Cover dish and let crumbs heat while the food carryover cooks.
• Good on casserole and potato dishes.
• I occasionally will sprinkle a bit on a buttered vegetable to add a bit of character.

GARLIC BREAD

24 servings
1 serving equals
1 bread exchange
1 fat exchange
115 calories
C-15   P-2   F-5

1 loaf sliced French bread
$^1/_4$ teaspoon garlic powder
$^1/_2$ cup soft butter or margarine

In a small bowl mix the softened butter or margarine with the garlic powder. Open the bread and assemble on a piece of paper toweling twice as long as the loaf. Spread 1 teaspoon of the garlic mixture on each piece of bread. Wrap in the paper towel and micro on high 2–2$^1/_2$ minutes. Let rest 2–3 minutes for internal steam to completely melt the butter.
• Take care not to overheat or bread will toughen and be very dry when cooled.
• If a more "flavorful" garlic bread is desired, increase the garlic powder to taste.

EASY DUMPLINGS

Serves 8
1 serving equals
$3/4$ bread exchange
milk exchange negligible
55 calories
C-12 P-2 F-0

1 cup buttermilk biscuit mix (Bisquick type)
$1/3$ cup skim milk

Mix milk and biscuit mix until smooth. Drop by heaping teaspoons on broth or stew, making 8 dumplings. Cover and cook on high 3 minutes. Rotate $1/4$ turn and continue cooking 2–3 minutes or until dumplings are cooked. Let rest covered 2 or 3 minutes before peeking.

The microwave makes perfect dumplings as they remain snowy white.

RICE

Serves 4
1 serving equals
1 bread exchange
$1/4$ fat exchange
82 calories
C-15   P-2   F-1.5

1 cup rice
1 teaspoon salt
1 teaspoon butter or margarine
2 cups water

In a 3 quart glass casserole or batter bowl (sounds big but rice really expands and bubbles up) combine all ingredients. Cover with plastic wrap, making a dent in the wrap with your hand before tightening around top. This allows for growth room as the steam cooks the rice and this helps prevent boiling over. Microwave high 7 minutes, stir and re-cover. Cook an additional 6–7 minutes. Let set covered 10 minutes before serving.
• Cooked rice will stay hot about 20 minutes.
• Refrigerate leftovers as rice reheats well.

COMPANY RICE

Serves 4
1 serving equals
$1/2$ fruit exchange
$1/4$ fat exchange
1 bread exchange
115 calories
C-20   P-2   F-1.5

1 small apple, peeled and diced
$1/2$ cup unsweetened orange juice
$1/2$ cup water
1 teaspoon butter or margarine
$1/2$ teaspoon salt
$1/2$ teaspoon cinnamon
$1^1/3$ cups instant rice

Combine first seven ingredients in $1^1/2$ quart casserole. Cover and micro on high 3–4 minutes, stirring once. When liquid comes to a full boil stir in rice and cover tightly. Let rest 7–8 minutes. Stir after resting 5 minutes and quickly replace the cover.
• I like this with ham for a change of pace.

INSTANT RICE

Serves 4
1 serving equals
$1/4$ fat exchange
1 bread exchange
85 calories
C-15   P-2   F-1.5

1 cup water
$1/2$ teaspoon salt
1 teaspoon butter or margarine
1 cup instant rice

In a 1 quart casserole combine water, salt and butter or margarine. Micro covered on high 2–3 minutes until water comes to a full boil. Remove from oven, add rice and stir to mix. Cover tightly and let rice rest 7–8 minutes. Stir at 5 minutes and quickly re-cover.

MOCK RICE PILAF

$1/2$ cup cooked rice equals
1 bread
70 calories
C-15   P-2   F-0

• For a change of pace, omit salt and butter and add a beef or chicken bouillon cube to the water before adding rice. Cook as above. Season as desired after cooking.

CORN ON THE COB

2 Servings
1 serving equals
70 calories
1 bread exchange
C-15   P-2   F-0

2 small ears corn

Choose nice fresh corn with tight husks. Remove all outer husks leaving about a two leaf layer around the kernels and silk. Arrange the corn on a paper towel on the bottom of the oven. In the husk covering, microwave on high 2 minutes. Rotate ears $^{1}/_{4}$ turn and continue cooking 2 minutes. Let rest with the husks on for 5 minutes to carryover and steam through. Corn will be sweet, tender and juicy.

Season as desired but remember the cob area will hold the heat so will be hot inside at first.

Popped corn is a super snack. Check with your micro manufacturer for directions on popping fat-free corn in your oven. 3 cups of popped corn equal 1 bread exchange, 70 calories, C-15, P-2 F-0. Sprinkle with favorite seasoning and enjoy! (I am leery of the paper bag method of popping corn as a bag can catch on fire and ruin your oven.)

SPICY CABBAGE RELISH

Makes 4 cups
$1/2$ cup serving equals
$1/2$ fat exchange
1 vegetable exchange
48 calories
C-5   P-2   F-2.5

4 teaspoons butter or margarine
2 cups finely shredded cabbage
1 medium green pepper, chopped
1 small onion, chopped
2 medium tomatoes, chopped
2 tablespoons wine vinegar
2 teaspoons prepared mustard
1 teaspoon Worcestershire sauce
$1/2$ teaspoon salt
$1/4$ teaspoon hot Tabasco type pepper sauce
$1/8$ teaspoon pepper

Place butter or margarine in glass 2 quart casserole. Place in micro and cook on high until melted—about 45 seconds. Add remaining ingredients to butter and mix well. Cover and microwave on high 7–9 minutes, stirring after 4 minutes. Serve hot over hot dogs, with Polish ring or your favorite sausage. Refrigerate leftovers and use hot or cold.
• If cooking sausage—remember to prick and let steam escape.

ORIENTAL GREEN BEANS

Serves 4
1 serving equals
1 vegetable exchange
$1/4$ fat exchange
37 calories
C-5   P-2   F-1.5

1 package (9–10 oz.) frozen French cut green beans
1 tablespoon water
2 tablespoons minced fresh onion
1 can (4 oz.) sliced mushrooms
1 tablespoon soy sauce (may use more to taste)
1 tablespoon slivered almonds

Combine green beans, water and onion in 1 quart glass casserole. Cover and cook 4 minutes on high stirring once. Drain mushrooms. Stir in soy sauce and mushrooms. Cover and heat on high 1–$1 1/2$ minutes. Sprinkle on slivered almonds.
• May be served with additional soy sauce if desired.
• If you like a softer vegetable, substitute canned green beans (16 oz.) drained, and use bean juice for water.

MUSHROOMS IN WINE

Serves 2
1 serving equals
1 vegetable exchange
1 fat exchange
75 calories
C-5   P-2   F-5

$^1/_2$ pound fresh mushrooms
   (or 8 oz. can drained)
2 teaspoons butter
$^1/_2$ teaspoon seasoned salt
$^1/_4$ teaspoon granulated garlic powder
2 tablespoons dry wine

    Clean and slice mushrooms. Melt butter in microwave and add mushrooms and seasonings. Cover and cook on high 2 minutes. Add wine and cook an additional minute or until tender. Let rest 2–3 minutes for flavors to marry. Serve hot with steak or roast.
• Bits of beef stir fry cooked with the mushrooms and wine makes a delicious quick meal. You may need to increase the seasonings if beef strips are added.

PICKLED BEETS

Serves 4
1/2 cup equals
1 vegetable exchange
25 calories
C-6

1/4 cup water
1/3 cup vinegar
1/4 teaspoon salt
1/4 teaspoon ground cloves
1 can (about 2 cups) diced or sliced beets
artificial sweetener equal to 1/2 cup sugar

Drain beet juice into 1 quart casserole. Mix water, vinegar, salt and cloves with juice and cook on high about 3 minutes until mixture comes to a full boil. Stir twice during cooking to distribute the heat. Remove from the oven and add beets and cover tightly to carryover cook 5 minutes. Stir in the sweetener and refrigerate. Serve cold as a vegetable or relish.
• These are good alone or mixed in a green salad.
• My favorite beets to use are crinkle cut as they give an interesting look to an everyday type food.

FRESH VEGETABLES

Vegetables follow a basic rule of 6 minutes on high per pound. Simply clean vegetables, rinse and place in a glass dish with whatever water remained on the vegetable after rinsing. Cover tightly (I prefer plastic wrap) and cook. Take care in removing the plastic wrap after cooking as there will be much hot steam escaping.

- For softer veggies add 1 tablespoon water per pound.
- Check exchange list for amounts per serving.
- Microwaved fresh vegetables make a non-vegetable eater return for seconds.
- Solid vegetables like acorn squash and potatoes must have vent holes poked in them with a knife or fork on all sides to allow steam to escape . . . or they may burst.
- Place thickest part of vegetable toward the outside of the dish or with uniform veggies like asparagus alternate vegetables end for end. This helps insure evenly cooked tender vegetables.

GREEN BEANS WITH BACON AND ONION

4 servings
1 serving equals
1 vegetable exchange
1/4 fat exchange
35 calories
C-5   P-1   F-1

1 (16 oz.) can sliced or cut green beans
1/2 slice bacon
1 tablespoon chopped sweet onion
salt and pepper to taste

Cut bacon into small bits and place in 1 quart casserole with onion. Micro high 1 minute to cook bacon and onion bits. Stir and add canned beans. Cover and heat 6 minutes, stirring once. Let rest covered 3–4 minutes before serving.

- A small can of drained mushrooms added with the beans make a nice special occasion vegetable. Add 1 1/2–2 minutes to the cooking time, stirring twice. With mushrooms the recipe still equals the same values as listed above for a half cup serving.
- We thoroughly enjoy the beans as a "hot salad" occasionally and will top drained beans with a teaspoon of ranch type salad dressing.

• I often serve special "bean sauce" (the ranch or a dill ranch dressing) to company to dress up the vegetable and the beans become something special. The small amount of dressing does not make the beans cool rapidly as it is added by each person on their own serving at the table. A teaspoon of ranch dressing has the same value as sour cream or yogurt—whichever you use as your base.

<u>COOL CARROTS</u>

Serves 4
1 serving equals
$\frac{1}{2}$ fruit exchange
$\frac{1}{2}$ vegetable exchange
33 calories
C-8   P-1   F-0

1 package (4 serving) sugar free orange gelatine
2 cups water
1 cup drained canned pineapple
   (crushed in own juice is best)
1 cup grated fresh carrot

Drain pineapple and reserve juice to be included in the 2 cups liquid. Micro on high the orange gelatine and one cup of water 2 minutes, stirring 3 times to dissolve gelatine. Pour into 1 quart mold and stir in the pineapple, carrot and remaining cup of liquid (water and drained pineapple juice). Refrigerate until firm.

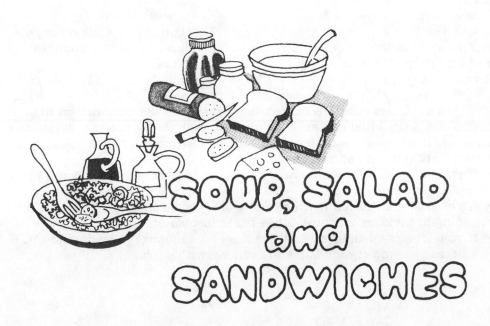

SOUP, SALAD and SANDWICHES

CLAM CHOWDER

1 strip bacon, diced
1/3 small onion chopped
1 small potato, peeled
  and diced
2 cups skim milk
salt and pepper to taste
1 can (4 oz.) clams

Serves 2
1 serving equals
1 fat exchange
1/2 bread exchange
1 cup skim milk exchange
2 low-fat meat exchanges
270 calories
C-20   P-23   F-11

In a 1 quart casserole saute bacon and onion 2–3 minutes on high. Add potato, clams and clam liquid and cook on medium high (80%) power 5–6 minutes, stirring twice. Add milk and seasonings and heat on medium high 3–4 minutes, stirring twice, until hot but not boiling. Let rest 3–4 minutes before eating.

• If you have leftover bits of crab, shrimp or any cooked seafood add them for a seafood chowder.
• If you desire a thicker chowder add a bit of cornstarch or flour to the milk before adding to the clam mixture. Stir 4 times instead of twice.
• If your diet can handle an additional 1/4 fat exchange (12 calories) add 1/4 teaspoon butter to the top of each cup and sprinkle with paprika.

CHICKEN VEGETABLE SOUP

1/4 cup cooked chicken, chopped
1/3 cup finely chopped carrot
1/3 cup finely chopped onion
1/3 cup finely chopped celery
1 cup chicken broth
1 cup skim milk
1 1/2 tablespoons flour
2 tablespoons water
salt and pepper to taste

Serves 4 (3/4 cup)
1 serving equals
1/2 vegetable exchange
1/4 milk exchange
1/4 low-fat meat exchange
bread—negligible
50 calories
C-9 P-5 F-1

Place finely chopped vegetables and chicken stock in a 2 quart glass bowl or casserole. Micro high covered with plastic wrap 4–5 minutes until vegetables are tender, stirring twice. Add milk and chicken. Mix flour in water to form thin paste and stir into "soup." Micro on medium high (80%) uncovered about 3 minutes, stirring each minute until slightly thickened. Let rest 5 minutes covered. Season with salt and pepper.

• A tablespoon of pimento is also good in the chicken soup and will not change the values.

TOMATO BOUILLON

Serves 4
1 serving equals
1 vegetable exchange
25 calories
C-5 P-0 F-0

2 cups tomato juice
1 can consomme (chicken or beef)
¹/₂ bay leaf, if desired
dash of sauterne, if desired
salt and pepper to taste
lemon slices
parsley flakes

In a 2 quart casserole combine consomme and tomato juice, and bay leaf if used. Micro on high 3–4 minutes uncovered until broth comes to a boil, stirring twice. Remove from oven. Take out bay leaf and discard. Add dash of sauterne and salt and pepper to taste. Pour into mugs and top with a slice of lemon. Sprinkle parsley flakes for garnish, if desired. Let set 3–4 minutes uncovered before drinking.

It's warm and a great fill'er upper not fill'er outer.

• This also makes a rather nice warm appetizer.

CREAM OF POTATO SOUP

2 cups peeled, diced raw potatoes   Serves 8
2 cups chicken broth   1 serving equals
2 strips bacon, diced $1/2$ fat exchange
$1/4$ cup finely chopped onion $1/2$ bread exchange
6 cups skim milk $3/4$ milk exchange
salt and pepper to taste   120 calories
dash of nutmeg   C-17   P-16   F-5

    Place chicken broth in a 3 quart casserole and micro on high covered 3 minutes. Add potatoes, cover and cook on high 4–5 minutes, until potatoes are tender. Remove and let rest while onion and bacon cooks. Place onion and bacon in small pie plate and cook on high 2–3 minutes, stirring once. Bacon should be crisp and onion soft. Add bacon, onion and drippings to stock mixture. Stir in milk and season to taste. Heat on medium high (80%) power to desired temperature taking care not to boil.
    Enjoy!
• This is good served with open-faced sandwiches or a tossed salad.

CREAMY SEAFOOD SOUP

Serves 8
1 serving equals
$1/2$ fat exchange
1 low-fat meat exchange
$1/2$ bread exchange
$3/4$ cup milk exchange
175 calories
C-17   P-23   F-7

Make cream of potato soup and add 2 cups cooked, shrimp, crab, clams, salmon or white fish or a combination with the milk. Heat through, stirring often, taking care not to boil.
• Freeze leftover dabs until you collect 2 cups of the mixed seafood. Makes a nice ''on hand'' type meal and good use of bits of leftovers.

OYSTER STEW

Serves 6
1 serving equals
2 low-fat meat exchanges
1/2 milk exchange
1/2 fat exchange
173 calories
C-6   P-18   F-8.5

1 pint small oysters
3 cups skim milk
1/2 teaspoon salt
1/4 teaspoon pepper
1 tablespoon Worcestershire sauce (optional for zip)
1 tablespoon butter or margarine
paprika for garnish

In a 2 quart glass casserole heat oysters on high in their liquid 1 minute. Add milk and heat 3–4 minutes stirring twice on medium high (80%) power. Add seasonings and cook 1 minute until desired temperature, taking care not to boil. Let rest a minute or two and drop 1/2 teaspoon of butter on top of each serving and sprinkle lightly with paprika.

CRAN-APPLE SALAD

Serves 8
1 serving equals
$1/4$ fruit exchange
vegetable exchange negligible
12 calories
C-3   P-0   P-0

2 cups low calorie cran-apple juice cocktail
1 (4 serving) envelope sugar free orange gelatin
1 cup chopped apple (with peeling)
$1/2$ cup chopped celery

Micro on high 1 cup of the juice and gelatin $1^1/_2$ minutes stirring once. Remove from micro and stir well to make sure all gelatin is dissolved. Add remaining juice and chill until about the consistency of egg white. Stir in apple and celery. Pour into 1 quart mold or make in 1 quart casserole and cut into squares. The red/green combination is pretty if served on a lettuce leaf.

This is a good wintertime salad and is especially nice with poultry or ham.

FRUIT SALAD DRESSING

Makes about $3/4$ cup
1 tablespoon equals
8 calories
exchanges negligible
C-2

1 egg
dash of salt
1 tablespoon flour
1 tablespoon unsweetened orange juice
$2/3$ cup unsweetened pineapple juice
artificial sweetener to equal $1/3$ cup sugar

Beat egg in 2 cup glass measuring cup. Add one half of the pineapple juice and flour and mix well to form a smooth paste. Add salt and stir in remaining juices. Micro on medium high (80%) power 3–4 minutes, stirring 3 times until thickened. Let rest 3 minutes uncovered and stir in sweetener. Chill and serve with any fruit salad or top fruit cups.
• One recipe of dressing will make enough fresh fruit salad to fill both halves of a pineapple shell. Really good with fresh pineapple to serve in individual "boats" at a luncheon.

FRUIT CUP

$^1/_2$ cup equals
40 calories
1 fruit exchange
C-10   P-0   F-0

Fresh fruit is colorful, tasty and refreshing, and makes a nice mixture in a bright dish or fruit "bowl" (watermelon rind, cantaloupe shell, pineapple skins work well for a group or cut the oranges in half and save the peel for individual fruit cups).

Apples, oranges, berries, grapefruit, nectarines, peaches, pears, pineapple or tangerines equal 1 fruit exchange in $^1/_2$ cup servings. These may be mixed.

Serve chilled topped with Fruit Salad Dressing.

The fruit is also excellent served on a fresh fruit tray or large platter with the Fruit Salad Dressing in the center as a dip.
• I always take a large fruit tray to potlucks and buffets and often am asked to bring one to parties where everyone brings an appetizer—with the fruit "dip."

SPRINGTIME SPINACH SALAD
(One of our very favorites)

Serves 5
1 serving equals
1 vegetable exchange
$1/2$ medium-fat meat exchange
$1/2$ fat exchange
72 calories (with dressing)
C-5   P-5.5   F-4

Salad
1 bunch fresh spinach
2 slices bacon, crumbled
2 hard cooked eggs, chopped
1 slice sharp cheddar cheese diced or 1 ounce sharp cheddar grated ($1/4$ cup)
Dressing
$2/3$ cup vegetable oil
$1/3$ cup ketchup
$1/3$ cup red wine or tarragon vinegar
$1/3$ cup chopped sweet onion
2 teaspoons Worcestershire sauce
artificial sweetener to equal $1/3$ cup sugar

91

Dressing: Mix all ingredients in a covered jar. Shake to mix and refrigerate at least 2 hours before serving.
• Makes enough dressing for 3 salads. Keep remaining dressing refrigerated.
Salad: Wash spinach leaves and pat dry. Break into bite size pieces and set aside. Micro bacon on high until crisp (approximately $1\frac{1}{2}$ minutes), drain and crumble. I usually prepare the eggs as baked eggs in muffin papers (no oil needed) until hard cooked. Place spinach in large bowl and top with egg, cheese and bacon bits. Just before serving shake dressing well and pour over salad to moisten and toss lightly until well mixed. Salad also is good served on individual salad plates with the dressing on the side.
• I usually bake the eggs at the same time I make the dressing so they can cool thoroughly (see page 38).
• For a light luncheon entree double the egg and cheese so the salad equals 1 vegetable exchange, 1 medium-fat meat exchange, $\frac{3}{4}$ fat exchange and 135 calories per serving. Hearty appetites can consume double portions as a meal so double the values, and enjoy with a hot roll. Makes a nourishing and light meal.

VICKY'S CROQUE MONSIEUR
(Yummy open-faced sandwiches)

Serves 3
1 serving equals
1 high-fat meat exchange
1 bread exchange
1 low-fat meat exchange
$^1/_3$ medium-fat meat exchange
250 calories
C-15   P-18   F-13

6 (1 oz.) slices ham
1 egg, beaten
$^3/_4$ cup grated Swiss cheese
1 teaspoon dry sherry
$^1/_2$ teaspoon parsley, snipped
dash garlic salt
3 slices French bread, toasted (my preference is sour dough so I cut it in half to toast)
dash of nutmeg to garnish

   Arrange toast on micro proof plate. Top with ham. Combine remaining ingredients in a small dish and spoon mixture over meat. Micro on high covered 1$^3/_4$ minutes until cheese melts and sprinkle lightly with nutmeg if desired.
• This is also tasty with slices of chicken or turkey breast exchanged for the ham. Values remain the same.
• I really enjoy this accompanied with fruit cup and dill pickle spear.

CHRISTOPHER COLUMBUS
(A favorite of Carrie for brunch)

Serves 4
1 sandwich equals
$1/4$ vegetable exchange
1 low-fat meat exchange
1 high-fat meat exchange
230 calories
C-17   P-16   F-11

2 English muffins, toasted (4 halves)
4 slices cooked ham or Canadian bacon (1 oz. each)
12 broccoli flowerettes
1 recipe quick cheese sauce (page 59)

    Wash and trim broccoli, shake off excess water and place in glass pie plate covered with plastic wrap. Micro high $2^1/_2$–3 minutes until fork tender. Prepare cheese sauce. Pop muffins in toaster while making sauce. Layer toasted muffin with ham, broccoli and top with sauce on individual serving plates. Micro on high about 45 seconds to heat thru. Sprinkle with paprika, if desired.
• These are also good with asparagus spears exchanged for the broccoli. Directions and values remain the same.

"TOASTED" CRAB AND CHEESE SANDWICHES

2 servings
1 serving equals
2 low-fat meat exchanges
1 fat exchange
$^3/_4$ high-fat meat exchange
2 bread exchanges
370 calories
C-30   P-24   F-17

4 ounces crab meat
2 teaspoons mayonnaise
dash of salt and pepper
4 slices sandwich bread, toasted
2 slices processed cheese ($^3/_4$ oz. each) American type

Mix crab and mayonnaise. Add salt and pepper. Divide mixture and place on 2 slices of bread. Top each with cheese and remaining bread. Micro on medium high (80%) power wrapped in a paper towel $1^1/_4$–$1^1/_2$ minutes until cheese is melted and crab warm. Let rest 2–3 minutes.

TOASTED TUNA AND CHEESE SANDWICHES: use rye or wheat toast and exchange like amounts of tuna and cheddar for the crab and American processed cheese. Values and directions are the same.

OPEN FACED SOURDOUGH SEAFOOD SANDWICHES

1 cup crab or shrimp,
  cooked or a combination
1/4 cup diced celery
2 tsp. finely chopped
  green onion or chives
1 cup shredded cheddar
  cheese (4 oz.)
8 teaspoons mayonnaise
4 whole (8 halves) sourdough
  English muffins, toasted

8 sandwiches
1 serving equals
1 low-fat meat exchange
1/2 high-fat meat exchange
1 fat exchange
1 bread exchange
220 calories
C-15   P-13   F-12

Toast muffins. Combine seafood, celery, onion and cheese. Add mayonnaise, a dash of salt and pepper if desired and blend. Spoon equally on halved sourdough muffins. Place in a glass baking dish that has been lined with a paper towel and micro on high 1 minute uncovered. Turn 1/4 turn and cook an additional 1/2–1 minute. Check to see if filling is warm and cheese is melted. If they need more oven time—zap them 15 seconds at a time, taking care not to overcook as overcooking will toughen the muffin.

Salmon sandwiches: substitute cooked (canned works well) salmon for the shell fish. With salmon I often add a chopped dill pickle when I mix the filling. Same values.

TUNA MELT

Serves 4
1 serving equals
1¹/₂ low-fat meat exchanges
1¹/₂ fat exchanges
1 high-fat meat exchange
1 bread exchange
310 calories
C-15   P-20   F-20

4 slices cheddar cheese
1 can (6¹/₂ oz.) tuna in water
2 tablespoons mayonnaise
dash of onion powder
4 English muffin halves, toasted
4 tomato slices, if desired

Drain tuna fish and mix with mayonnaise. Season to taste with onion powder. Place one-fourth of the tuna mixture on each muffin half, add tomato slice if desired, and top with cheese slice. Place on a paper towel on baking dish or rack in micro and cook on high 1¹/₂–2¹/₂ minutes until cheese is melted and beginning to bubble. Let rest 3–4 minutes before eating.

• Also super on rye or sourdough toast slice. Same values as with muffin half if one slice of bread is used.

TOASTED CHEESE SANDWICHES
(NO FAT ADDED!!)

Serves 1
Per sandwich equals
1 high-fat meat exchange
2 bread exchanges
240 calories
C-30   P-11   F-8

1 slice cheese
2 slices bread, toasted (white, wheat, rye or a combination of varieties)

Toast bread in conventional toaster. Place cheese between toast slices. Place sandwich on a paper towel to prevent a soggy bottom and micro on high 25–30 seconds to melt cheese. Let rest 2–3 minutes before biting into as cheese really holds heat!
• If your bread is starting to get dry, toast it and put in the freezer for use in toasted sandwiches. It's ready when you are and better to use it for yourself than for bird food!

MEAT AND CHEESE SANDWICHES: 1 ounce (usually slice) of the following meats are really good with the toasted cheese and increase the value to include 1 low-fat meat exchange—55 additional calories and C-0 P-7 F-3.

Ham, roast beef, pastrami or corned beef (lean only).
Cheese may be your choice: American, cheddar, Swiss, etc.

MOM'S SPECIAL

Serves 1
1 serving equals
1 high-fat meat exchange
1 bread exchange
1 fat exchange
215 calories
C-15   P-9   F-13

1 slice tomato
1 strip bacon, halved
$\frac{1}{2}$ English muffin, toasted
1 slice cheddar cheese

     Cook bacon on high 30 seconds on a paper plate. Layer muffin with tomato, cheese and partially cooked bacon to top it off. Micro high on a paper towel 30–40 seconds until cheese is bubbly and bacon cooked. Let rest 2–3 minutes before eating as heat holds inside.
• This is also good on rye or pumpernickel toast.
• Makes a nice change of pace for breakfast too!
It's warm and chewy . . . almost like having a pizza.

HAMBURGERS

Serves 5
1 serving equals
2 medium-fat meat exchanges
2 bread exchanges
290 calories
C-30   P-18   F-11

1 pound extra lean ground meat
5 hamburger buns or 10 slices
    bread

Free garnishes as desired: lettuce, mustard, onion slice, dill pickle slices, tomato slice.

Divide meat into 5 equal portions approximately $1/3$ inch thick. Arrange patties on a bacon rack or plate lined with a paper towel. The rack will drain off the fat—the towel will absorb it. Both methods reduce calories and improve meat flavor. Cover with waxed paper. Micro on high as directed in chart for the first side. Turn and micro as for second side. Let rest covered with waxed paper 1–2 minutes to carryover cook. Check for doneness. The gray color will disappear as meat browns but surface will not be crusty. Any meat with natural fat will brown in the microwave.

Patties	First side	Second side
2	$1^1/_2$ minutes	$3/_4$–1 minute
5	2 minutes	1–2 minutes

HOT DOGS

Serves 1
Per serving
1 high-fat meat exchange
2 bread exchanges
240 calories
C-30   P-11   F-8

1 hot dog bun
1 weiner
mustard, as desired

Spread bun with mustard. Place weiner in bun and wrap in paper towel. Cook on high for 45–50 seconds for 1 hot dog, 1–1¼ minutes for 2 hot dogs.
- When buying hot dogs check to see if the weiners are approximately one ounce. In these days of inflation often the packages have been reduced to 12 ounces from a pound and still contain the same number of weiners . . . only they have gotten "skinny." If the weiners are less than an ounce add ¼ slice of cheese in the bun before heating and values remain the same.
- If you are allowed more meat exchanges—cheese dogs are delicious. Split a slice of cheese and place one half slice on each half of the bun before inserting weiner. When heated cheese will melt and hold the dog together. Add 1 high-fat meat exchange to the basic hot dog and 100 calories—C-0   P-7   F-8 for cheese.

OLÉ DOGS

Serves 4
1 serving equals
1³/₄ bread exchange
1 medium-fat meat exchange
1¹/₄ high-fat meat exchange
¹/₂ fat exchange
350 calories
C-27 P-20 F-18

1 can (16 oz.) chili with beans
4 weiners
4 tortillas
¹/₄ cup shredded cheddar cheese
¹/₄ chopped onion

Place tortillas in micro on high wrapped in a paper towel for 30 seconds. Remove from oven and place 2 tablespoons chili on each tortilla, place weiner in center and roll up; place seam sides down in glass baking dish. Cover roll-ups with remaining chili. Heat, covered, on high 7–8 minutes. Remove from micro, top with cheese and onions. Cover and let rest 5 minutes before serving.

Good with green salad and a fresh fruit plate.

TACOS

1 pound extra lean ground beef
1 package (Lawrys) taco
  seasoning mix
1/2 cup water
8 tortillas
1 cup shredded cheddar cheese
2 cups shredded lettuce
1 chopped tomato (if desired)
chopped fresh onion (if desired)

8 tacos
1 taco equals
1 bread exchange
1/2 high-fat meat exchange
1 1/2 medium-fat meat exchange
raw veggies are free
235 calories
C-15   P-17   F-12

Brown meat and pour off fat. (Can be browned in a plastic collander and fat will automatically drain off as meat cooks.) Mix meat with seasoning mix and water in a 2 quart casserole and micro on high 2 minutes. Stir and reduce power to medium (60%) and cook covered 5 minutes. Let rest while heating tortillas, 4 at a time, for 30 seconds on high wrapped in a paper towel. Place meat, cheese, lettuce and tomatoes in shell evenly and top with chopped onions as desired.

Olé!

TOSTADO

Makes 8
Same calculations as TACO
plus ½ additional high-fat meat
exchange, 50 calories, C-0   P-3.5   F-4
if ¼ cup cheese is used on tostado

Sauce
1 cup equals
1 bread exchange
70 calories
C-15   P-2   F-0
2 tablespoons equal
9 calories
C-2   P-0   F-0

 Cook meat as directed for tacos with seasonings. Heat tortilla and lay flat.
Spoon on meat, ¼ cup shredded cheese and top with about 1 cup shredded lettuce
and chopped tomatoes.
 For a nice sauce drizzle with Contadina tomato sauce (just plain for mild sauce)
or with a few drops of tabasco hot pepper sauce mixed in for a hotter sauce.
• TACO SALAD: Make tostado in a bowl without the tortilla and deduct 1 bread
 exchange, 70 calories, C-15 P-2 F-0 from the taco calculations.

MAIN DISHES

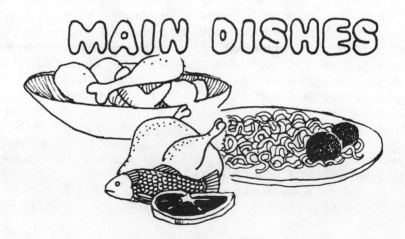

EASY BEEF ROAST

1 ounce cooked equals
1 low-fat meat exchange
55 calories
C-0   P-7   F-3

My favorite roasts in the microwave are boneless, uniform shaped, and tender cuts like rump, (rolled and tied) rib eye, top round and tip.

To cook, pierce meat with tip of knife and insert garlic pieces, if desired. Place on microwave rack (or 2 inverted micro proof saucers) in a microwave dish. Your bacon rack is perfect for a small roast as it will easily collect the juices for gravy.

Cook the roast on high and turn the roast over half way through estimated cooking time. Generally rare to medium roasts are the most popular. Degree of doneness is best determined by using a microwave thermometer, a conventional meat thermometer used OUTSIDE the oven or the oven food probe. Temperature is more accurate than time for determining doneness. However, if you don't have a thermometer a general guide is 6 minutes to the pound for medium meat.

The roast will brown naturally because of its fat content in 10–15 minutes. If you desire a browner roast, simply baste with soy sauce, Worcestershire sauce or a small amount of Kitchen Bouquet.

Remove roast from the oven, cover and allow to rest 10 minutes to seal in juices before carving. The roast will increase 10–15° during standing time.

De-fat drippings and use for gravy, freeze to add to soup stock later or make au jus for sandwiches when roast is to the leftover stage.

Gravy is always most popular at our house and is a favorite of men . . . especially with mashed potatoes.

Temperatures for Roast Beef

	Out of the oven	Cutting temperature
Rare	120°	135°
Medium rare	130°	145°
Medium	140°	155°
Medium well	150°	165°
Well done	160°	175°

• Cutting temperature is after 10–15 minutes of covered standing time.

POT ROAST WITH VEGETABLES
(one pan dinner)

1 2 pound beef chuck roast (boneless
   or about 2$^{1}/_{2}$ pounds with bone—
   remove bone before cooking roast)
1 teaspoon salt
$^{1}/_{4}$ teaspoon pepper
5 carrots, peeled
5 potatoes, peeled
5 small onions OR 1 large quartered
1 tablespoon flour

Serves 5
1 serving equals (lean meat only)
4 medium-fat meat exchanges
1 vegetable exchange
1 bread exchange
1 fat exchange
440 calories
C-20 P-32 F-27

Mix flour, salt and pepper in a bag. Trim meat and shake in flour bag to coat. Place in baking dish or micro roaster with 1 cup of water and the onion. Micro on high covered tightly for 10 minutes. Turn roast over, re-cover and micro on medium power (50%) for 30 minutes. Rotate roaster $^{1}/_{4}$ turn, add carrots and potatoes. Re-cover and cook on medium an additional 30–35 minutes. Rest covered (without lifting the lid so the vegetables will steam) 10 minutes to complete carryover cooking. Serve with meat juices that have been skimmed and thickened. To thicken juices mix 2 teaspoons cornstarch (or flour) in 1 tablespoon cold water and stir into juices after meat and vegetables have been removed. Micro high 2–3 minutes stirring each minute.

• The fat exchange is added as there is fat accumulated in the juices that is absorbed by the veggies and is in the gravy . . . and what's a pot roast without potatoes and gravy?

New England Boiled Dinner . . .
CORNED BEEF AND CABBAGE
A one pot meal!

Serves 6
1 serving equals
4 medium-fat meat exchanges
2 vegetable exchanges
1 bread exchange
420 calories
C-25 P-34 F-22

4 cups water
3 pounds corned beef round
6 small potatoes, pared
6 small carrots, pared
6 wedges cabbage (1 head)

In a 3 quart casserole or micro roaster cook water on high 2 minutes covered. Add meat and juices from the meat sack and cover. Micro on high 30 minutes. Turn meat over and rotate the pan $1/4$ turn. Re-cover and continue cooking on high 30 minutes. Add potatoes and carrots, re-cover and micro high 12–16 minutes. Turn vegetables over, add cabbage, re-cover and cook on high 10–14 minutes. Let carry-over cook covered 8–10 minutes. Remove meat and test vegetables for tenderness. If necessary cook any vegetables not done enough 3–4 minutes while slicing the meat. Slice the meat in thin slices across the grain.

- Corned beef will shrink.
- Makes super leftover sandwiches . . . especially with melted Swiss cheese on toasted rye!
- 2 tablespoons drained sauerkraut, corned beef and Swiss cheese make a mock reuben on toasted rye. See page 98 for calculations and directions. Kraut is free.

BEEF STEW

Serves 4
1 serving equals
3 low-fat meat exchanges
$1^1/_4$ bread exchanges
1 vegetable exchange
275 calories
C-21 P-25 F-9

2 cups water
1 pound boneless beef cubes
4 small potatoes, quartered
3 carrots, peeled and cut in
   1″ pieces
1 medium onion, quartered
salt and pepper to taste
2 tablespoons frozen peas,
   if desired
2 tablespoons flour

      In a 3 quart casserole combine beef, $1^1/_2$ cups water, onion, and carrots. Cook on high covered 6–7 minutes. Reduce heat to low (25%) and add potatoes. Cook on low covered for 55–60 minutes until vegetables are all tender. Stir twice during cooking. Add peas. Mix flour with remaining water and stir into stew. Blend well and cover. Cook on low 7–8 minutes until gravy is thickened, stirring twice. Let rest 5 minutes before serving.

• Super topped with easy dumplings. Add dumplings at the time you add the thickening for the gravy.

• May add more water if a thinner broth is desired.

SWISS STEAK

1 pound tenderized round steak
1 can onion soup in beef broth
$1/3$–$1/2$ can water
1 tablespoon flour
4 pared carrots, if desired

Serves 4
1 serving equals
3 low-fat meat exchanges
$1/2$ bread exchange
$1/2$ fat exchange
225 calories
C-8   P-22   F-11.5
With carrots add
1 vegetable exchange
25 calories
C-5   P-2   F-0

Cut meat into four servings and trim off fat. Coat meat with flour by shaking in a paper sack. Arrange in an 8×8 glass baking dish or 2 quart casserole and top with soup and water. Cover with vented plastic wrap and micro high for 10 minutes. Re-arrange meat and add carrots, if desired. Re-cover and micro on medium (50%) for 25–35 minutes. Meat and carrots should be fork tender. Let rest 10 minutes tightly covered to finish carryover cooking and tenderize a bit more.

• If desired you may thicken the juices after removing the meat. Mix 1 tablespoon cornstarch in 2 tablespoons cold water. Stir into the juice, micro on high 2–3 minutes stirring each minute until thickened.

MEAT LOAF

1 pound extra lean ground beef
1/4 cup cracker crumbs
1 egg
1/2 cup tomato or V-8 juice
1/4 cup finely chopped onion
1 teaspoon salt
1 teaspoon garlic salt
1 teaspoon Worcestershire sauce
2 tablespoons ketchup (optional)

Serves 4 (generously)
1 serving equals
3 medium-fat meat exchanges
1/4 vegetable exchange
1/4 bread exchange
250 calories
C-5   P-22   F-16.5

Combine all ingredients except ketchup and pack into a glass ring mold or 9 inch glass pie pan and use a custard cup to make center to form a ring. Cook on high for 3 minutes, rotate 1/4 turn and cook for 3 additional minutes. Pour ketchup on top and cook for 5 more minutes rotating once for even cooking. Let rest about 5 minutes to firm up. Remove drippings and serve. Excellent hot or cold.
• May use dry bread crumbs for cracker crumbs.
• Don't remove drippings during cooking or meat loaf will be dry. Extra lean meat has very little waste.

INSTANT MEAT LOAF
Quick to prepare . . .
shelf to oven time . . .
about 2 minutes

2 pounds extra lean ground beef
2 large eggs
1 can (8 oz.) tomato sauce
2 tablespoons instant minced onion
2 tablespoons parsley flakes
1 teaspoon Worcestershire sauce
1 teaspoon Italian seasoning
2/3 cup instant oatmeal
1/2 teaspoon pepper
1 teaspoon salt
2 tablespoons ketchup

Serves 8
1 serving equals
1/2 bread exchange
3 medium-fat meat exchanges
1/4 vegetable exchange
265 calories
C-10   P-22   F-16.5

Combine all ingredients in large mixing bowl, except ketchup. Mix well. (If you have short fingernails you can put all ingredients in a plastic bag to mix and you don't even have the bowl to wash.) Place in 2 quart glass ring mold or 10 inch pie pan with a custard cup in the center to form a ring. Cook uncovered on high for 14 minutes. At 7 minutes remove excess juice and fats (oatmeal will have absorbed enough juice to keep moist) and turn 1/4 turn. Top with ketchup and continue cooking remaining time. Pour off any excess fat at the end of the 14 minute time and cover. Let rest about 7 minutes to firm before serving.

BASIC MEATBALLS
Serve alone or with favorite sauce

Serves 4
1 serving equals
3 medium-fat meat exchanges
$1/4$ bread exchange
245 calories
C-4   P-21   F-16.5
(Per serving: 3 large or 5 small meatballs)

1 pound lean ground beef (15% fat)
1 egg
$1/4$ cup chopped onion
$1/4$ cup dry bread crumbs
1 teaspoon salt
$1/2$ teaspoon garlic powder
1 teaspoon Worcestershire sauce
$1/8$ teaspoon pepper

    Mix all ingredients together and form meatballs. This will make 12 (about 2 inch balls) or 20 ($1^1/2$ inch balls). Place on bacon rack or in a circle in a large pie plate. Micro high 4–5 minutes. Rotate dish $1/4$ turn and continue cooking 3–4 minutes or until desired doneness. Meatballs will brown and firm up while standing, so be careful not to overcook. Let rest 5 minutes covered with waxed paper.

MOM'S SAUCY MEATBALLS

Meatballs
1 pound ground beef (15% fat)
1/4 cup onion, chopped
1/4 cup cracker crumbs
3–4 tablespoons skim milk
1 teaspoon salt
1/8 teaspoon pepper
1/4 teaspoon poultry seasoning
Sauce
1 can cream of mushroom soup
3/4 cup hot water
Garnish
chopped parsley

Serves 4
1 serving equals
3 medium-fat meat exchanges
3/4 bread exchange
1 fat exchange
330 calories
C-12   P-22   F-21.5
Serves 6
1 serving equals
2 medium-fat meat exchanges
2/3 fat exchange
1/2 bread exchange
215 calories

Meatballs: Mix all ingredients together and form meatballs. Place on rack or in a circle in a large pie plate and micro high 4 minutes. Drain off grease and put meatballs in casserole. Mix soup and water and pour over meatballs. Cover and cook on high power about 10 minutes stirring and rotating 1/4 turn half way through cooking time. Meatballs should be tender and moist with a bubbly sauce. Let rest 4–5 minutes before serving. Garnish with chopped parsley if desired.
• Super with noodles or rice.

CHILI

Serves 4
1 serving equals
3 medium-fat meat exchanges
1 vegetable exchange
1 bread exchange
320 calories
C-17   P-25   F-16.5

1 pound extra lean ground beef
1/4 cup chopped onion
1/2 cup chopped green pepper
1 clove garlic, minced OR 1/4 teaspoon garlic powder
1-2 tablespoons chili powder
1 teaspoon salt
1 can (16 oz.) tomatoes, not drained
1 can (16 oz.) kidney beans, not drained

In a 2 or 3 quart casserole, brown the meat on high about 6 minutes, with onion, green pepper and garlic. Pour off all fat half way through cooking time, stir and continue cooking remaining time. At the end of the cooking time, pour off any additional fat. Mix with remaining ingredients and cook 12-15 minutes, stirring twice. Let rest about 5 minutes covered before serving.

• The first step may be done in a micro proof collander and grease will drip out as meat, onion and pepper cook. Stir three times during 6 minute cooking time.

TERIYAKI KEBOBS

Teriyaki Sauce
(Free food)
1 cup soy sauce
2 cloves crushed garlic
1 teaspoon dry mustard
1½ teaspoons ground ginger
artificial sweetener to equal
   1 teaspoon sugar

Serves 6
1 serving equals
2 low-fat meat exchanges
1 vegetable exchange
135 calories
C-5   P-16   F-6

Sauce: combine all ingredients in a jar with a tight lid. Shake and refrigerate. Sauce will keep several weeks so make the whole recipe and use it on steak, chicken or ribs. Sauce is a free food—Enjoy!

Kebobs
1 green pepper
1 pound lean beef cubes
12 small boiling onions
12 cherry tomatoes
12 mushrooms
½ recipe teriyaki sauce

Wash cubes and marinate in teriyaki sauce 4–6 hours. Wash pepper, remove seeds and cut in 1 inch sections. Peel onions and clean mushrooms. Arrange meat cubes on skewers (non metal—bamboo work well) alternating with mushrooms, green pepper and onions. Place on rack and baste with sauce. Microwave on high 3–4 minutes, turning once. Baste again after turning. DO NOT overcook. Let rest 2 minutes. Serve with tomatoes on end of skewers. Really good in hot weather.

TERIYAKI CHICKEN

2 whole chicken breasts
   (about ½ pound each)
½ recipe teriyaki sauce

Serves 4
1 serving equals
3 low-fat meat exchanges
165 calories
C-0   P-21   F-9

Cut chicken breasts in half lengthwise and bone them if desired. (I always ask the butcher to bone them.) Marinate in sauce 2–3 hours. Place on rack, cover with waxed paper and cook on high 2–3 minutes. Turn chicken over, baste and cook covered an additional 2–3 minutes. Check chicken for doneness. Let rest 5 minutes before serving. Chicken will continue cooking during rest period. Temperature, thickness and with or without bones will vary cooking time. Chicken pieces may also be used in kebobs and are a popular change of pace.

EASY CHICKEN RICE SUPPER

1 cup uncooked rice
1 teaspoon salt
1 can cream of chicken soup
1 can warm water
2 pounds chicken parts
  (our preference is the breast)
2 carrots, peeled and
  cut in half (if desired)

Serves 4
1 serving equals
1/2 fat exchange
1 1/4 bread exchanges
3 low-fat meat exchanges
280 calories
C-19   P-24   F-11.5
With carrot add per serving
1/2 vegetable exchange
12 calories
C-3   P-0   F-0

In a 3 quart microwave casserole mix salt, rice, carrots, soup and water. Place chicken parts, thick side out, around outside of casserole and baste with a bit of the liquid. Cover tightly and cook on high 20 minutes. Shake casserole to stir. Don't lift cover, cook on high an additional 10–15 minutes. Let carryover cook covered 10 minutes. Check for doneness. Cook another minute or two covered if needed.

• If small chicken parts are used or chicken is room temperature, decrease cooking time accordingly.
• If cover is plastic wrap prick a small hole in one corner to allow a bit of a vent or pressure will loosen cover.

CHICKEN CACCIATORE

Serves 4
1 serving equals
3 low-fat meat exchanges
$1/2$ bread exchange
vegetable exchange negligible
200 calories
C-8   P-22   F-9

2 chicken breasts halved (8 oz. each) or 1 $2^{1/2}$ pound chicken
1 (15 oz.) can tomato sauce
4 ounces mushrooms, sliced
$1/2$ medium onion, chopped
1 teaspoon oregano
1 teaspoon salt
$1/4$ teaspoon garlic powder
$1/4$ teaspoon pepper

Place chicken in 8 × 8 baking dish (if a whole chicken is used—use a dish appropriate for one layer of chicken). Mix all other ingredients and pour over chicken. Cover with waxed paper and micro high 9–10 minutes. Re-arrange chicken and re-cover with wax paper and cook 6–10 minutes or until chicken is tender. Rest 8–10 minutes covered to carryover cook.
• This is really tasty served with cooked spaghetti noodles.

CRISPY CHICKEN

Serves 6
4 low-fat meat exchanges
3/4 bread exchanges
milk exchange negligible
265 calories
C-12   P-29   F-12

3 pounds chicken pieces (I usually use quartered breasts)
1 cup cornflake crumbs
1/2 teaspoon onion salt
1/2 teaspoon garlic salt
1 teaspoon paprika
pinch of oregano or poultry seasoning (if desired)
1/2 cup skim milk

Remove skin from chicken pieces, rinse and drain. Combine cornflake crumbs and seasoning in a plastic bag. Dip chicken pieces (usually 2 at a time) in milk and shake in the crumb bag to coat. Arrange chicken pieces in baking dish with large parts to the outside. (Wings, legs and small parts in the center.) Cover loosely with plastic wrap. Cook on high 18–20 minutes, rotating 1/4 turn once, until chicken is desired doneness.

• Any leftover crumbs I sprinkle over the chicken as I feel my diet has been "charged" for it.

STEWED CHICKEN

Chicken serves 4
1 serving equals
3 low-fat meat exchanges
165 calories
C-0   P-21   F-9

1 cut up fryer (2½–3 lbs.)
1 can chicken broth
salt and pepper to taste
1 soup can water

Place chicken, broth, water and seasoning in large casserole with glass cover. Cook on high, covered, 10 minutes. Reduce power to medium (60%) and continue cooking covered 20 minutes or until chicken is very tender. If desired make dumplings on broth while chicken is in the pan. For a gravy broth may be thickened with a flour and water paste after removing chicken and dumplings. Check index for dumpling recipe.
• Leftovers are great for sandwiches and salads.
• Broth may be frozen and later used for soups or gravy.

SIMPLE POT PIE

2 cups cut up cooked chicken
  or turkey
1 can cream of chicken soup
1 package (10 oz.) mixed vegetables,
  thawed
$1/2$ cup milk
$1/8$ teaspoon pepper
$1/8$ teaspoon salt
dash poultry seasoning, if desired
1 (8 oz.) can refrigerator biscuits
parsley flakes, optional

Serves 4
1 serving equals (without biscuits)
2 low-fat meat exchanges
$1/4$ bread exchange
$1/2$ fat exchange
1 vegetable exchange
200 calories
C-9 P-17 F-8
Biscuits add per biscuit
1 bread exchange
70 calories C-15 P-2 F-0

    In a 2 quart casserole dish combine all ingredients except biscuits and parsley flakes. Microwave high 9–10 minutes covered, stirring twice during cooking time. Arrange biscuits evenly in a ring around the edge of the casserole and sprinkle with parsley flakes, if desired. (I sprinkle as it gives biscuits some color.) Cook on high 3–4 minutes uncovered rotating dish once. Rest covered 5 minutes. Biscuits will be cooked but soft—somewhat dumplinglike.

SAUCY PORK CHOPS
(One of our favorites)

Serves 4
1 serving equals
3 medium-fat meat exchanges
1/2 bread exchange
1 fat exchange
305 calories
C-7.5   P-22   F-21.5

4 (4 oz.) loin pork chops, fat removed
1 can cream of chicken soup
4 tablespoons ketchup
1/2 teaspoon onion powder
1/4 teaspoon pepper
2 tablespoons Worcestershire sauce

Place pork chops in corners of glass skillet or large baking dish. Combine soup, ketchup, Worcestershire sauce, pepper and onion powder. Pour over chops. Cover and cook on high 8 minutes. Turn 1/4 way and cook 6 more minutes until pork chops are done. Rest covered about 10 minutes before serving. Serve with sauce.
• Excellent served with rice.

WEINER SCHNITZEL

Serves 4
1 serving equals
4 low-fat meat exchanges
$1/2$ high-fat meat exchange
1 bread exchange
$3/4$ fat exchange
375 calories
C-15   P-34   F-19

4 veal cutlets (about 4 oz. each) pounded thin
2 thin slices cooked ham, halved (1 oz. each)
2 slices Swiss or Jack cheese (1 oz. each) halved
1 cup seasoned dry bread crumbs
$1/2$ teaspoon salt
dash of allspice
1 egg, beaten with 2 teaspoons skim milk
3 teaspoons butter or margarine

Lay cutlets flat. On one side of each cutlet place $1/2$ slice ham and $1/2$ slice cheese. Fold over and secure with a wooden toothpick. Mix crumbs with salt and a dash of allspice and roll cutlet in crumbs. Dip in egg-milk mixture and reroll in crumbs. Melt 2 teaspoons of the butter or margarine in an 8×8 glass pan and place schnitzel in dish. Pat approximately $1/4$ of the remaining butter on each schnitzel.

Cook about 8 minutes on medium power (60%) covered with wax paper, turning after 5 minutes. Let carryover cook 5 minutes covered with waxed paper. Check veal at earliest time (when turning) and adjust final cooking time. Veal is low fat and is best not overcooked. Garnish with lemon slices and parsley.
• Boneless chicken breasts may be substituted for veal cutlets.

BAKED HAM WITH PINEAPPLE

2 pound ham
  serves 8
1 serving equals
3 low-fat meat exchanges
1/4 fruit exchange
175 calories
C-3 P-21 F-9

• Fully cooked hams only have to be heated to serving temperature—130° internal temperature. Canned hams heat more rapidly than pre-cooked "regular" hams because of their uniform size and flat shape.

2-3 pounds cooked ham
1 small (4 slice) can unsweetened pineapple
pinch of cloves
1/4–1/2 teaspoon dry mustard
paprika

Drain pineapple and reserve juice. Place ham in flat micro baking dish. Remove gelatin if ham is canned type. Mix juice with cloves and dry mustard. Pour over ham and top with pineapple rings. Micro on high 6 minutes per pound, rotating 1/4 turn after 6 minutes. Remove from oven and cover with waxed paper while it carryover cooks, about 10 minutes. Sprinkle with paprika.
• If you prefer firmer pineapple rings, place them on the ham at the time of rotation.
• If a meat thermometer is used be sure it is one made for microwave ovens or remove ham from oven and use thermometer outside the oven.

DEVILED CRAB OR SHRIMP

4 teaspoons butter or margarine
1 tablespoon finely chopped onion
2 tablespoons flour
$1/2$ teaspoon Worcestershire sauce
$1/2$ teaspoon dry mustard
$1/2$ teaspoon salt
$1/4$ teaspoon pepper
1 cup milk
2 cups crab, salad shrimp or a
   combination
$1/4$ cup grated cheddar cheese
$1/4$ cup bread crumbs

Serves 4
1 serving equals
1 fat exchange
$1/2$ bread exchange
$1/4$ milk exchange
2 low-fat meat exchanges
$1/4$ high-fat meat exchanges
235 calories
C-11   P-19   F-13

Combine butter or margarine and onion in 1 quart casserole and cook on high $1^{1/2}$–2 minutes. Stir in flour making a smooth paste. Add milk and stir until well blended. Cook on high 3–4 minutes stirring every minute until sauce is thick and smooth. Add seasonings and shell fish. Cover and cook 4–5 minutes, until heated through and bubbly on medium high (80%). Sprinkle with bread crumbs and cheese, cover tightly, and let carryover cook 5 minutes.

- This makes a pretty dish served in individual scallop shells.
- This is excellent served over toast points.

QUICK SEAFOOD NEWBURG

Serves 4
1 serving equals
(including toast or popover)
$1\frac{1}{4}$ bread exchange
2 low-fat meat exchanges
$\frac{1}{2}$ fat exchange
225 calories
C-19   P-16   F-8.5

1 (10 oz.) can cream of shrimp soup
1 tablespoon sherry
1 tablespoon skim milk
8 ounces cooked, shrimp, crab, lobster, scallops or a combination of shellfish
4 slices toast or 4 popovers
1 small (4 oz.) can of mushrooms, if desired

In a 1 quart casserole, mix undiluted soup, milk and sherry. Cook covered on high 3–4 minutes until hot and bubbly around edges. Stir and add the seafood. Cover and heat 2–3 minutes, stirring once to heat the seafood. Let rest 3–4 minutes covered. Serve on toast points or in popovers.

Drained mushrooms may be added with the seafood, if desired. Increase cooking time 1 minute and stir twice while heating. For the mushrooms add ¼ vegetable exchange, 6 calories.

• A tablespoon of chopped pimento offers a spark of color and is a nice flavor addition. Pimentos would be free.

VICKY'S FISH ALMONDÉ

Serves 8
1 serving equals
3 low-fat meat exchanges
1¼ fat exchanges
vegetable exchange negligible
220 calories
C-0   P-21   F-16

1 tablespoon butter or margarine
1/2 cup almond slivers
2 pounds fresh fish fillets (sole, snapper, cod)
1 cup combined fresh chopped vegetables (green pepper, onion, celery)
1 tablespoon butter or margarine
1 tablespoon lemon juice
salt and pepper to taste

In 8 x 8 glass dish combine 1 tablespoon butter and almonds. Cook on high for 3 minutes, stirring twice. While almonds cook, prepare vegetables in a small micro proof dish and add remaining 1 tablespoon of butter or margarine. Remove almonds from oven and cook little dish of vegetables on high 2 1/2 minutes. With a fork or slotted spoon remove almonds from dish. Coat fish with remaining butter in baking dish and arrange fish in baking dish with the large pieces to the outside of the dish. Sprinkle with lemon juice and salt and pepper. Top with vegetables. Cover with waxed paper and cook on high 8 minutes. Sprinkle with almonds, re-cover and cook 1 additional minute. Let rest 4–5 minutes before serving.
• This recipe is a favorite shared by ODA's own Vicky Hutchinson.

SALMON LOAF

Serves 4
3 low-fat meat exchanges
1 bread exchange
¼ milk exchange
255 calories
C-18   P-25   F-9

1 (16 oz.) can salmon, drained
soft bread crumbs (centers of 4 slices)
1 cup thin white sauce
1 egg
1 tablespoon lemon juice

Make the white sauce and set aside while you tear the bread into crumbs and take the skin and large bones out of the salmon. Mix the egg and lemon juice into the white sauce and beat the mixture with a fork until blended. Add to salmon and bread crumbs and fold until well mixed. Pour into one quart glass ring mold. Micro on high 7 minutes. Remove and cover with waxed paper for 5 minutes for salmon loaf to carryover cook. Garnish with lemon slices and paprika.

CRISPY FISH

Serves 4
1 serving equals
3 low-fat meat exchanges
$1/2$ fat exchange
$1/4$ bread exchange
205 calories
C-4   P-21.5   F-11.5

1 pound fish fillets
1 cup cornflakes
2 teaspoons butter or margarine
1 teaspoon lemon juice (optional)

Crush cornflakes in a plastic bag. Melt the butter or margarine in glass pie pan 1 minute on high. Add lemon juice. Roll fish in butter to coat. Lemon in the butter gives a much fresher flavor. Shake in crumbs and arrange the fish on bacon rack (thickest part toward the outside edges) and micro high 4–6 minutes, turning dish $1/4$ turn after 2 minutes. Fish generally is cooked at the earliest time and should flake easily, but not be dry. Serve with additional lemon wedges.

DILLY SALMON OR HALIBUT STEAKS

4 salmon or halibut steaks (about
   4 oz.) each of 2 large salmon or
   halibut steaks, halved
1/2 cup finely chopped celery
1/2 teaspoon parsley flakes
1/2 teaspoon salt
1/2 teaspoon dill weed
1/2 teaspoon pepper
1/4 cup white wine
4 teaspoons butter or margarine

Serves 4
1 serving equals
1 fat exchange
3 low-fat meat exchanges
210 calories
C-0   P-21   F-14

     On high power combine celery, butter, parsley, salt, dill and pepper and cook 2–3 minutes until celery is tender. Stir in the wine and add salmon or halibut with the narrow ends toward the center of the dish. Heat covered with waxed paper 5–6 minutes rotating the dish 1/4 turn after 3 minutes. Let carryover cook, covered 3–4 minutes before serving. (Check to see if fish flakes easily, if not zap on high covered one additional minute.)

SCALLOPS IN LEMON BUTTER

Serves 4
1 serving equals
$1^1/_2$ fat exchanges
3 low-fat meat exchanges
235 calories
C-0   P-21   F-16.5

1 pound scallops, fresh or thawed
2 tablespoons butter or margarine
pinch of basil
pinch of crushed rosemary
$^1/_4$ teaspoon salt
2 tablespoons lemon juice
paprika

On high power melt butter or margarine in glass dish (I use an 8 inch round cake pan) with rosemary, basil and salt 1 minute. Add scallops and lemon juice and stir well to coat. Reduce heat to medium (60%) power. Cover with wax paper and cook 7–8 minutes until scallops are tender and white. Stir twice during cooking time. Sprinkle with paprika, cover with wax paper and let carryover cook 5 minutes. Serve and enjoy.

• Take care not to overcook scallops or they will become rubbery and tough.

SKINNY FISH FILLETS

Serves 4
1 serving equals
3 low-fat meat exchanges
165 calories
C-0   P-21   F-9

1 pound fish fillets (or steaks)
1 lemon

Drizzle lemon juice on fish and cover with plastic wrap. Cook on high 4–6 minutes turning dish half way through cooking time $1/4$ turn. Cook with thickest part of fish toward outside of baking dish. Rest 4 minutes.
- Fish generally cooks in 4 minutes per pound because it does not have connecting tissue.
- This is a super way to fix fish to be used at a later date or in another recipe calling for cooked fish.

SAUTEED SHRIMP

Serves 4
3 low-fat meat exchanges
1$\frac{1}{2}$ fat exchanges
235 calories
C-0   P-21   F-16.5

2 tablespoons butter or margarine
$\frac{1}{2}$ teaspoon garlic powder
$\frac{1}{2}$ teaspoon poupon (wine) mustard
1 tablespoon dry white wine
2 teaspoons parsley flakes
1 teaspoon lemon juice
1 (12 oz.) package frozen, peeled and deveined shrimp

In a one cup measuring cup (glass) melt butter or margarine on high about 1 minute. Stir in garlic powder, mustard, wine, lemon juice and parsley flakes. Heat an additional 15 seconds. Separate shrimp and place in 9 inch glass cake pan. Pour butter mixture evenly over shrimp and stir to coat. Cover tightly with plastic wrap and microwave on high 4–7 minutes, stirring every 2 minutes until shrimp are opaque. Let rest, covered, 1$\frac{1}{2}$–2 minutes. Serve with remaining butter mixture in individual ramekins or on toast points. Also good served with rice.
• These also make nice appetizers . . . serve with napkins.

COQUILLE ST. JACQUES

Serves 6
1 serving equals
2 low-fat meat exchanges
$1/2$ bread exchange
1 fat exchange
190 calories
C-8   P-15   F-11

1 pound fresh scallops (or frozen scallops, thawed)
1 cup dry sherry
$1/2$ bay leaf
$1/2$ pound fresh mushrooms, sliced
2 tablespoons butter or margarine
1 tablespoon lemon juice
2 tablespoons diced onion
$1/2$ teaspoon salt
$1/8$ teaspoon pepper
$1^{1/2}$ tablespoons flour
Topping
$1/4$ teaspoon paprika
dash cayenne, optional
1 tablespoon Parmesan cheese
3 tablespoons bread crumbs

On medium (60%) power, cook scallops covered with ¼ cup of the sherry and the bay leaf for 5–6 minutes until scallops are tender and white. Stir once during cooking. Drain liquid off scallops and reserve ¼ cup. Discard bay leaf. In a 1 quart glass measuring cup heat the butter, onion and mushrooms one minute, stir in flour, salt and pepper. Gradually add the remaining wine, reserved ¼ cup broth and lemon juice stirring until smooth. Cook 3–3½ minutes until mixture is thickened, stirring every minute. Pour over scallops, cover and heat 1–2 minutes until hot through still on medium power. Sprinkle with topping and let rest covered 3–4 minutes before serving.

• This is really nice served in individual scallop shells. Pour into individual shells before adding topping. Micro 15 seconds if necessary to heat the topping.

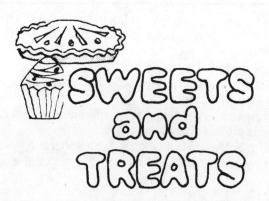

SWEETS and TREATS

JIFFY FRUIT JEL

Contains:
2 cups fruit juice
Check exchange list for
portion size for 1 fruit
exchange for type of
juice used in recipe
1 fruit exchange equals
40 calories
C-10 P-0 F-0

2 cups fruit juice
1 envelope unflavored gelatine

Make your own gelatine for salads and desserts by heating one cup of fruit juice in micro until boiling. While juice boils dissolve the gelatine in the cool cup of juice. Remove from micro and stir until completely mixed and all gelatine crystals have dissolved. Refrigerate until firm.
- This has super flavor and servings are equal to the amount of juice allowed for the variety of juice used.
- Artificial sweetener may be added to taste, if desired, after the gelatine has completely dissolved.
- For a dessert top with a tablespoon of real whipped cream that has been artificially sweetened, add 23 calories, $1/2$ fat exchange and F-2.5 for the whipped cream.

FREE JIFFY JEL

Free Food
calories and exchanges
negligible
CPF-0

Free gelatine may be made quickly using two ingredients and following the Jiffy Fruit Jel directions on preceding page.

1. Substitute sugar free diet soda for the fruit juice. Flavor remains the same as the soda and since the sweetener has already been added and heated previously there will not be any change in the flavor from an aftertaste of artificial sweetener.

2. Substitute unsweetened drink powder (Kool-Aid type) mixed with water to equal the fruit juice. Let the mixture rest 3 minutes after completely dissolving the gelatine and sweeten to taste with artificial sweetener.

• For a stiffer Jel dissolve the gelatine in the cup of liquid that is heated in the microwave dissolving during cooking. Stir after liquid and gelatine have been in the micro on high 1 minute.

STRAWBERRY TOPPING

Makes about 2½ cups
¼ cup equals
½ fruit exchange
20 calories
C-5   P-0   F-0
2 teaspoons are free

2 envelopes unflavored gelatine
1 can sugar free strawberry soda
1 teaspoon lemon juice
2 cups strawberries
artificial sweetener to equal 2 tablespoons sugar, if desired

Mix gelatine and soda in a 2 quart casserole (keeps splatters at a minimum) and micro on high 2 minutes, stirring once to dissolve gelatine. Add lemon juice and strawberries and cook on medium (50%) 3–4 minutes. Berries will be soft and juicy, but not mushy. Crush berries with potato masher. Let set uncovered 3–4 minutes, stirring twice before adding sweetener.

- I like it best warmed slightly for pancakes or waffles because it gets a little runny.
- This topping is great on toast, cheesecake, pancakes, waffles, ice cream or just off the spoon.
- This will keep in the refrigerator about a week.

SAUCY APPLE SAUCE

Serves 2
1 serving equals
$^1/_2$ fat exchange
1 fruit exchange
65 calories
C-10   P-0   F-2.5

1 cup apple sauce
1 teaspoon butter or margarine
cinnamon and nutmeg to taste
1 drop red food coloring, if desired

Combine all ingredients. Micro on high about 1 minute until butter melts and apple sauce is just warm. Stir and use warm to top pancakes, waffles or for a change on hot oatmeal.
• If a sweeter sauce is desired, add artificial sweetener, to taste, after removing warm sauce from the microwave.

BAKED APPLES
(For breakfast, snacks or dessert)

Serves 5
1 serving equals
1 fruit exchange
40 calories
C-10   P-0   F-0

5 small apples
1 can sugar free creme soda
$1/2$ teaspoon cinnamon

Wash and core apples and make a slit in the skin for a vent about $3/4$ of an inch from the top all around the apple. Mix soda and cinnamon. Place apples in a circle in a glass cake or pie pan. Pour soda in center of apples and cover with wax paper. Cook on high 4–6 minutes rotating $1/4$ turn at 2 minutes. Prick apples with fork to test for doneness. Let rest at least 5 minutes before serving. Refrigerate any "leftovers." Good warm or cold.
- A bit of red food coloring mixed in the soda gives a rosy look.
- About 3 raisins dropped in each center before cooking adds flavor and a bit of variety.
- Garnish with whipped topping if used for dessert.

LEMON OR LIME SHERBET

Serves 5 (large servings)
1 serving equals
$^1/_2$ milk exchange
40 calories
C-6 P-4 F-0

1 envelope unflavored gelatine
$1^1/_2$ cups water
$^1/_2$ cup lemon or lime juice
1 tablespoon grated lemon or lime rind
$2^1/_2$ cups skim milk
artificial sweetener to equal $^3/_4$ cup sugar
food coloring, if desired

In a two quart casserole mix water and gelatine. Cook on high $1^1/_2$ minutes until water boils and gelatine is dissolved, stirring twice. Stir in juice and rind. Refrigerate about one hour. Add milk, sweetener and coloring. Mix well and freeze until partially frozen—approximately $1^1/_2$ hours. Beat with mixer until smooth. Pour into container and freeze and enjoy.
• If frozen in individual half cup dessert dishes or as dixie cups for the kiddies divide the above values in half.

147

GRAHAM CRACKER PIE CRUST

Serves 6
1 serving equals
1 bread exchange
1 fat exchange
115 calories
C-15   P-2   F-5

12 graham crackers (squares)
2 tablespoons butter or margarine
artificial sweetener to equal 2 tablespoons sugar (dry)

Place butter in glass 8 or 9 inch pie pan and micro on high for 30–45 seconds o melt. Crush graham crackers in a plastic bag with rolling pin. Mix cracker crumbs and sweetener with butter and press mixture firmly into sides and bottom of pie plate to form shell. Heat 1 minute on high to set crust. Cool completely before filling.

PASTRY CRUST
(one crust pie)

6 servings
1 serving equals
1 bread exchange
2 fat exchanges
160 calories
C-15   P-2   F-10

148

1 cup flour
¹/₃ cup shortening
2 tablespoons very cold water
dash of salt

     Mix flour and salt in small bowl. Add shortening and cut into flour until about the size of peas. Add water and mix into a ball. Roll out on lightly floured pastry canvas. Line glass pie pan with crust. (Will make an 8 or 9 inch shell.) Prick entire crust with a fork to make vents and prevent bubbling. Bake on rack at 80% power for 5–6 minutes rotating ¹/₄ turn at three minutes.

- For a crust with a browner color substitute cold diet cola for the water.
- May roll out thin and make two 8 inch shells. Thin shells cook in the minimum time.
- If cooked on full power, rotate ¹/₄ turn at 2 minutes and only cook 4–6 minutes.
- Lining the crust with waxed paper and setting a smaller glass plate inside will sometimes be helpful to prevent the crust from bubbling up and shrinking. Cook as directed. Remove the liner and waxed paper carefully before cooling so steam can escape and crust will be crisp not soggy.

FRUIT YOGURT PIE

Serves 6
1 serving equals
(with crust from preceding page)
$1/6$ milk exchange
$1/2$ fruit exchange
1 bread exchange
1 fat exchange
150 calories
C-22   P-3   F-5

1 graham cracker pie crust
1 8 ounce carton plain yogurt
1 cup raspberries, boysenberries, peaches or pineapple
1 cup prepared topping (Cool Whip type)

Wash and drain fruit. Squish one half cup of fruit with potato masher and stir into yogurt. Add remaining fruit and mix gently. Carefully fold in whipped topping. Pour into 8 inch graham cracker crumb crust and freeze until firm.

FROZEN YOGURT WHIP

Serves 6
1 serving equals
1/6 milk exchange
1/2 fruit exchange
C-7   P-1   F-0

1 8 ounce carton plain yogurt
1 cup raspberries, boysenberries, peaches or pineapple
1 cup prepared topping (Cool Whip type)

Wash and drain fruit. Squish one half cup of fruit with potato masher and stir into yogurt. Add remaining fruit and mix gently. Carefully fold in whipped topping. Pour into individual dessert dishes and freeze until firm.
• I often save 6 berries to garnish the top.
• If frozen in stemmed wine glasses the yogurt whip makes a festive light dessert.

PEACH MELBA

Serves 4
1 serving equals
$1/2$ fruit exchange
$1/2$ bread exchange
1 fat exchange
100 calories
C-13   P-1   F-5

4 small canned artificially sweetened peach halves (or canned without sugar)
4 $1/4$ cup scoops vanilla ice cream
4 teaspoons strawberry topping or artificially sweetened strawberry jam

In an 8 inch round pie plate micro peach halves cut side up $2^{1/2}$-3 minutes covered. Place in stemmed wine glasses (if you have them) and top with ice cream and topping. If you use the strawberry topping, two teaspoons are free, so I then like to put one teaspoon full in the center of the peach and the other on the top of the ice cream.

LIGHT LEMONY CHEESECAKE

Serves 12
including crust
1 serving equals
$3/4$ medium-fat meat exchange
$1^1/_2$ fat exchanges
$1/_2$ bread exchange
160 calories
C-8   P-7   F-9

1 graham cracker crust baked and cooled (page 148)

1 envelope unflavored gelatine
$3/4$ cup hot water
2 tablespoons lemon juice
2 packages (8 oz. each) cream neufchâtel cheese
artificial sweetener to equal $1/4$ cup sugar

In small glass mixer bowl dissolve gelatine in water on high about 1 minute, stirring twice. Remove from microwave. Open foil packages of cheese and place cheese in microwave about 45 seconds on high to soften. Combine all filling ingredients in the small bowl and beat with mixer until smooth. Pour into cooled crust and refrigerate until set, $1^1/_2$–2 hours.

- Top with crushed fresh fruit and a dollop of Cool Whip. 2 tablespoons fruit equals $1/4$ fruit exchange, 10 calories and adds C-2.5. 1 teaspoon Cool Whip is free.
- Bits of grated lemon rind are good in filling.
- More sweetener may be added if a sweeter cheesecake is desired.
- For a dessert tray it is fun to line muffin papers (12) with the crumbs on the bottom and bake as directed. Fill the individual "muffins" with cheesecake filling and unpeel individual little cakes before serving.
- Little tart papers (24) filled as above for muffins are very popular on an appetizer tray. I like to top these with a $1/2$ teaspoon of strawberry topping.
- Strawberry topping is particularly good on cheesecake.
- For a softer cheesecake filling increase water by 4 teaspoons in step one.

GUM DROP CHEWS

Free Food

1 can fruit flavored diet soda
1/2 cup lemon juice
1/2 teaspoon vanilla
5 envelopes unflavored gelatine
artificial sweetener to equal 1/4 cup sugar, if desired
food coloring for brighter festive chews

In a 1 cup glass measuring cup heat half the can of soda to the boiling point, about 2 minutes. Mix remaining ingredients with the other half can of soda in an 8 × 8 baking dish. Pour in boiling soda and stir until gelatine is dissolved. Refrigerate until firm. Cut into squares.

HOLIDAY TREATS:
Make above recipe using appropriate soda (example—orange for Halloween) and cut into holiday shapes with cookie cutters after mixture is firm.

FRUIT CHEWS:
Use 1 1/2 cups of fruit juice for soda. Divide into servings by type of juice used to equal 1/2 fruit exchange, 20 calories, C-5. Check exchange list for amounts of juice to equal one fruit exchange.

155

SPICY APPLE BUTTER

2 pounds cooking apples
2 tablespoons lemon juice
1 cup unsweetened apple juice
1/2 teaspoon cloves
1/4 teaspoon allspice
1 teaspoon grated lemon peel
2 tablespoons cider vinegar
artificial sweetener equal to
   1/4 cup sugar
2 tablespoons raisins (optional)

Makes 3 cups
1 tablespoon equals
7 calories
3 tablespoons equal
21 calories
1/2 fruit exchange
C-5 P-0 F-0

Wash, core and quarter apples, but leave peeling. In a 2 quart casserole or mixing bowl combine apples, juices and vinegar. Micro high, covered for 9-10 minutes until apples are soft. Stir every 2-3 minutes while cooking. Put cooked mixture through food mill or blender. Return to bowl and add remaining ingredients except sweetener. Cook on high 10-15 minutes, stirring every 2-3 minutes, until apple butter thickens. (I usually cook until no water seeps along the edges when a bit of the mixture is placed on a saucer.) Let rest 10 minutes before adding sweetener. Fill clean jars and refrigerate or freeze.

- If more sweetness is desired add more sweetener to taste. The tartness of the apples makes the amount of sweetener needed variable.
- If you like the flavor of cinnamon a bit may be added or you can exchange cinnamon to taste for the cloves and allspice. I prefer the stronger clove-allspice seasoning.

APPLE JELLY

Makes 1 cup
1 tablespoon equals
7 calories
3 tablespoons equal
21 calories
$\frac{1}{2}$ fruit exchange
C-5 P-0 F-0
$\frac{1}{3}$ cup equals
40 calories
1 fruit exchange
C-10 P-0 F-0

1 cup canned unsweetened apple juice
1$\frac{1}{4}$ teaspoon unflavored gelatine
1 teaspoon cornstarch
dash of salt
artificial sweetener to equal 1 cup sugar
1 tablespoon lemon juice

In a small (1 quart) mixer bowl mix the lemon juice, gelatine, salt and cornstarch until smooth with a wire whip. Add the apple juice and stir well. (At this point the mixture looks like dishwater, but it will clear up.) Micro uncovered on high for 5 minutes stirring each minute. Remove from oven and rest for 5 minutes before adding sweetener. Put in a 1 cup container, refrigerate and enjoy.

• Apple jelly mixed with a small amount of prepared mustard makes a nice sweet and tangy sauce for ham.

BLUEBERRY COMPOTE

Makes 2 cups
1 tablespoon equals
5 calories
exchanges negligible
2 tablespoons equal
$1/4$ fruit exchange
10 calories
C-5   P-0   F-0

1 package (10 oz.) frozen blueberries (unsweetened)
1 tablespoon lemon juice
$1^1/2$ teaspoons cornstarch
$1^1/2$ teaspoons unflavored gelatine ($1/2$ envelope)
dash of salt
artificial sweetener equal to 1 cup sugar

Partially thaw berries until you have about ¹/₂ cup of juice. In a 2 quart casserole mix lemon juice, berry juice, cornstarch, gelatine and salt. Micro high 1 minute to dissolve gelatine. Stir well. Add blueberries, mix well, cover and micro on high 3–4 minutes, stirring each minute until mixture comes to a full boil. Reduce heat to medium low (40%) and simmer along 2–3 minutes until mixture thickens a bit. Stir in sweetener after mixture rests 5 minutes. Pour into two 1 cup sterilized jars. Refrigerate. Keeps well in the refrigerator 3–4 weeks.

• This and a dollop of whipped cream makes restaurant style waffles at home!
• The dash of salt and lemon juice help cut the after taste of artificial sweeteners.
• Pour blueberry mixture into blender or strain it if a smoother-jam type is preferred. Do this while still warm and then reheat to a full boil to thicken again.
• Really good slightly warm to top ice cream or on cornbread.

FROZEN STRAWBERRY JAM
(Good to make year around)

Makes 3 cups
1 tablespoon equals
5 calories
free exchange

20 ounces frozen whole unsweetened strawberries
1 envelope unflavored gelatine
1/4 cup fresh lemon juice
1 tablespoon cornstarch
dash of salt
artificial sweetener to equal 1 1/2-2 cups sugar

In a 3 quart glass bowl thaw berries on high about 2 minutes. Squish with potato masher. In a separate bowl while berries are thawing, mix the lemon juice, gelatine, cornstarch and salt. Mix with berries, stirring well to blend. Microwave on high 4-5 minutes until mixture comes to a full boil. Stir and continue cooking on high 7-8 minutes more stirring 4 times. Test berries for doneness. Let rest 8-10 minutes and add the sweetener to taste. Food coloring may be added if desired. Without coloring jam is not as colorful as sugar sweetened products.

WORDS of WISDOM and INDEX

MILK

FATS

<u>MICRO SENSE . . . tried and true</u>

- Most foods (meats and vegetables) cook—done—on full power in 6 minutes to the pound. Fish is an exception as it cooks in 4 minutes to the pound as it does not have connecting tissue.
- For best results cook foods one dish at a time.
- To reheat food thoroughly, but not overcook, feel the bottom of the dish for temperature.
- Reheat food on same power level as it was cooked.
- If cooked covered—reheat covered.
- If cooked uncovered—reheat uncovered.
- Milk is best when reheated at 80% power.
- When doing a "plan over" meal—reheat foods in the same order as they were cooked.
- When defrosting: unwrap foods as a sealed wrapper holds steam and will begin cooking the food.
- Any food with a skin needs to be vented (examples: potatoes, squash, sausage).

- Any food that boils up (like rice) needs a container twice the size of the food.
- Foods with natural fat content (mainly meats) will brown in the microwave.
- Carryover cooking time is important to let the heat equalize. Food eaten too soon will burn!
- To only defrost half a meat item (hamburger for example) unwrap half and shield the other half with foil. Cut off defrosted portion and return frozen shielded part to freezer.
- Do not salt exposed foods—salt will dry and toughen. Salt also causes uneven cooking.
- Check a glass dish <u>without metal</u> for 30 seconds empty on high to see if it is micro proof—if it is HOT do not use it.
- Hot, steamy finger towels may be warmed on high 30 seconds.
- Ground beef cooked in a non-metal collander will be drained when cooked and ready for use. Place collander in a pie plate to simply collect the fat and grease.

- Place stale crackers in micro for a few seconds to make fresh and crisp.
- Use round dishes to prevent the overcooked corners that tend to occur in square cooking containers.
- Cover food as required to prevent drying and spattering.
- Stir the food or rotate the dish as directed during cooking to distribute the heat in the food as it cooks. Rotation should be a one-quarter turn to cook the food evenly.
- If you are unsure of a cooking time always undercook as you can cook an additional bit of time if necessary. Overcooked food is Hard, Tough, and Dehydrated and CANNOT be restored!
- Any plastic wrap works for a tight cover (anticipate hot steam when removing). Vent plastic wrap for lengthy cooking as the pressure will cause it to loosen.
- Wax paper covering allows some steam to escape.
- To hold food, cover with shiny side of foil inside to reflect heat and keep food warm longer.

• For best results, keep your oven clean. Spilled food absorbs energy.

Oven placement is important for best results. Here are microwave oven "floor plans" for placement of several items in the oven (example: baked apples, potatoes) or for placement in a cooking dish.

```
         X                    X X                       X
      one item              two items                X X
                                                  three items


            X X                          X
            X X                        X   X
         four items                    X   X
                                     five items
```

Soup, Salad and Sandwiches

Soups
Clam Chowder 82
Chicken Vegetable 83
Cream of Potato 85
Creamy Seafood Soup 86
Oyster Stew 87
Tomato Bouillon 84

Salads
Cran-Apple Salad 88
Fruit Salad Dressing 89
Fruit Cup 90
Springtime Spinach Salad 91
Taco Salad 104

Sandwiches
Beef and Cheese 98
Christopher Columbus 94
Corned Beef and Cheese 98
Hamburgers 100
Ham and Cheese 98
Hot Dogs 101
Mom's Special 99
Olé Dogs 102
Open Faced Sourdough Seafood 96
Pastrami and Cheese 98
Salmon Salad 96
Tacos 103
Toasted Cheese 98
"Toasted" Crab and Cheese 95
Tostado 104
Tuna Melt 97
Tuna and Cheese 95
Vicky's Croque Monsieur 93

Main Dishes

Beef

Basic Meatballs 115
Beef Stew 111
Chili 117
Corned Beef and Cabbage 109
Easy Roast Beef 106
Instant Meat Loaf 114
Meat Loaf 113
Pot Roast with Vegetables 108
Saucy Meatballs, Mom's 116
Swiss Steak 112
Teriyaki Kebobs 118

Chicken

Chicken Cacciatore 121
Crispy Chicken 122
Easy Chicken Rice Supper 120
Simple Pot Pie 124
Stewed Chicken 123
Teriyaki Chicken 119

Fish and Seafood

Crispy Fish 134
Coquille St. Jacques 139
Deviled Crab or Shrimp 129
Dilly Halibut 135
Dilly Salmon 135
Quick Seafood Newburg 130
Salmon Loaf 133
Sauteed Shrimp 138
Scallops in Lemon Butter 136
Skinny Fish Fillets 137
Vicky's Fish Almondé 131

Pork

Baked Ham with Pineapple 127
Saucy Pork Chops 125
Weiner Schnitzel 126

Sweets and Treats

Baked Apples 146
Free Jiffy Jel 143
Fruit Chews 155
Fruit Yogurt Pie 150
Frozen Yogurt Whip 151
Graham Cracker Pie Crust 148
Gum Drop Chews 155
Jiffy Fruit Jel 142
Lemon Sherbet 147
Light Lemony Cheesecake 153
Lime Sherbet 147
Pastry Crust 148
Peach Melba 152
Saucy Apple Sauce 145
Strawberry Topping 144

Jam and Jelly

Apple Jelly 157
Blueberry Compote 158
Frozen Strawberry Jam 160
Spicy Apple Butter 156